From the halls of Montezuma,
To the shores of Tripoli,
We fight our country's battles
In the air, on land and sea.
First to fight for right and freedom,
And to keep our honor clean;
We are proud to claim the title
Of United States Marine.

—First Verse of United States Marine Corps Hymn

Semper Fidelis—Always Faithful

—Motto of the United States Marine Corps

25 November 1998

Dear Mr. Flach,

I was delighted to receive a copy of your book, *The United States Marine Corps Workout.* After perusing its content, I can see the book will be a great guide for those who are readying themselves for recruit training or officer's candidate school, and fitness enthusiasts looking for a challenge or a varied workout. It is a welcome addition to my professional library. Your personal inscription makes it even more special.

Again, thank you for the book. I wish you the best in all of your future endeavors.

Sincerely,

C. C. KRULAK
General, U.S. Marine Corps
Commandant of the Marine Corps

Mr. Andrew Flach
The Hatherleigh Company
1114 First Avenue, Suite 500
New York, NY 10021

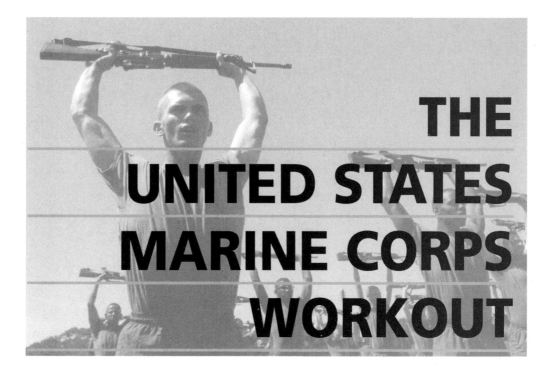

THE
UNITED STATES
MARINE CORPS
WORKOUT

RESEARCHED BY
ANDREW FLACH

PHOTOGRAPHED BY
PETER FIELD PECK

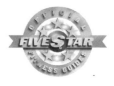

FIVE STAR FITNESS
NEW YORK

Five Star Fitness
An Independent Imprint of Hatherleigh Press

Five Star Fitness
1114 First Avenue, Suite 500
New York, NY 10021
1-800-906-1234
www.getfitnow.com

The use of the words United States Marine Corps, Marines, and USMC does not imply
an endorsement, either implicit or explicit, by the United States Marine Corps. This
publication has been authorized by the United States Marine Corps but is not an official
publication of the US Marines or Marine Corps Recruiting.

Before beginning any strenuous exercise program consult your physician. The
author and publisher of this book and workout disclaim any liability,
personal or professional, resulting from the misapplication of any of the
training procedures described in this publication.

A portion of the proceeds from the sale of each book
will be donated to the Navy-Marine Corps Relief Society.

All Five Star Publishing titles are available for bulk purchase, special
promotions, and premiums. For more information, please contact the manager
of our Special Sales Department at 1-800-906-1234.

ISBN: 1-57826-011-6

Cover design by Gary Szczecina
Text design and composition by DC Designs
Photographed by Peter Field Peck
with Canon® cameras and lenses on Fuji® print and slide film

Printed on acid-free paper
10 9 8 7 6 5 4 3

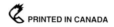

PRINTED IN CANADA

MISSION OF THE MARINE CORPS

THE MARINE CORPS SHALL:

• Be organized, trained and equipped to provide Fleet Marine Forces for service with the U.S. Fleet in the seizure or defense of advanced Naval bases and for the conduct of such land operations essential to the prosecution of a naval campaign.

• Provide detachments for service on armed vessels of the U.S. Navy and security detachments for the protection of property at Naval stations and bases.

• In connection with the Army, Navy and Air Force, develop the tactical techniques and equipment employed by landing forces in amphibious operations.

• Train and equip Marine forces for airborne operations in coordination with the Army, Navy and Air Force.

• Maintain four fully equipped and manned Divisions/Wings. Marine Regular forces shall comprise three of these Divisions/Wings. The fourth shall be the Marine Reserve.

ACKNOWLEDGMENTS

Thanks to the staff of the offices listed below for their contributions, which helped to make this book possible.

Marine Corps Public Affairs
Pentagon, Washington, DC
Captain Sean Gibson
Brigadier General Clifford L. Stanley

Marine Corps Base Parris Island, Public Affairs
Major Richard S. Long
Lieutenant Mark Brumfield

Marine Corps Base Quantico, Public Affairs
Major Paula Buckley
Captain Sean Clements

Marine Corps Recruit Depot San Diego, Public Affairs
Corporal Jerry Wright

Our editorial team: Susan Ruszala and Elizabeth Dilley
Our design and production team:
Dede Cummings and Gary Szczecina
Our logistics and support team: Kevin Moran and Bruce Slagle.
And to the many others who contributed to the success
of this mission: thank you!

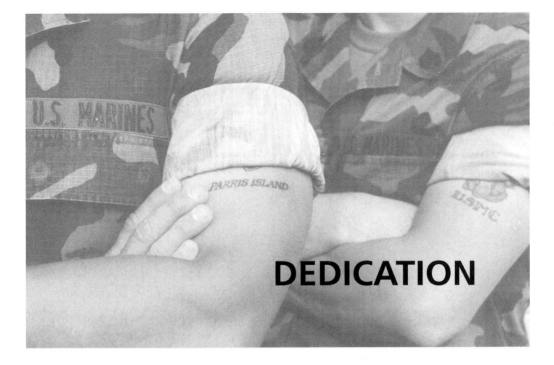

DEDICATION

This book is dedicated
to the Marine Corps Drill Instructors past and present,
those men and women whose efforts and inspiration turn
ordinary people into exceptional Marines.

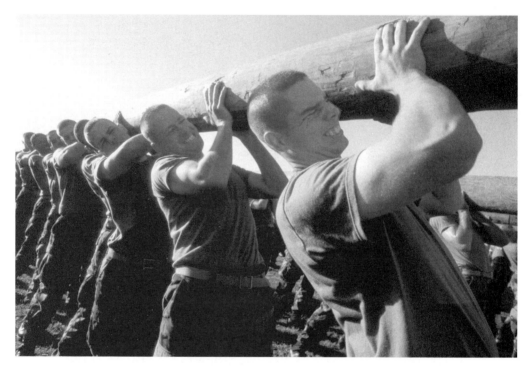

Log Drill Exercises, Parris Island.

CONTENTS

ABOUT THE SERIES

The Five Star Official Fitness Guides are designed to provide a fresh new perspective on the subject of personal health and fitness by documenting the physical training regimens of the United States Armed Forces.

To bring you this exciting information, we have shouldered our gear in the hot midday sun, on cold frosty mornings, in the dark of night. No workouts and training schedules were reorganized to meet our needs. Nor did we ask. We wanted to bring to you what's REAL. I like to think of these books as "fitness documentaries" —because that's what they are!

We have talked extensively with many individuals responsible for the physical fitness and welfare of the men and women of America's Armed Forces. We have discovered the most powerful workout and physical training routines in the world. We bring them to you with the hope that you will be inspired to value your health and pursue fitness activities throughout your life.

Wherever possible, primary source material is utilized. Documentation, interviews, briefs—all were assembled and culled for details and insights.

Important note: These books are not designed to be follow-to-the-letter workouts. That was never our intention. These books are a collection of information on the subject of fitness and physical training in the US military, full of techniques, routines, hints, suggestions, and tips you can learn from. Your workout should be individualized. We highly recommend you review your fitness plan with a certified trainer, coach, or other individual who possesses the proper knowledge to advise you in such a manner. And of course, consult your physician before commencing any new fitness program or before you intensify your current regimen.

Good luck and may lifelong fitness be your goal!

Andrew Flach
Peter Field Peck

SEMPER FIT!

Welcome to the Five Star Fitness look at Marine Corps training, the most ambitious undertaking so far in our series of military fitness books. Developed with the assistance and support of the U.S. Marine Corps, this book delivers the most accurate and up-to-date presentation of the physical fitness training programs unique to the Marines.

For those interested in becoming a Marine, we've included specific exercises and workout schedules designed to help you prepare for the rigorous fitness challenges that lie ahead. If you are content to remain a civilian, you'll discover one of the most convenient and simple—yet powerfully effective—approaches to physical fitness ever devised: The Marine Corps Daily 16. You'll learn that you can take your fitness program wherever you go. . .without equipment or the expense of a health club membership!

You'll notice that this book is structured in several parts. The first two parts document recruit fitness training and officer fitness training, with plenty of "real time" action, bringing you

> "Some people spend an entire lifetime wondering if they've made a difference to this world… the Marines don't have that problem."
>
> —President Ronald Reagan, 1985

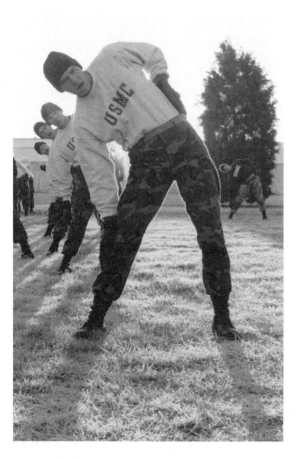

to the very places where men and women train to be Marines. Later in the book we detail workout plans designed to get you in great shape.

Throughout the book, we've included profiles of some of the remarkable individuals we met as we journeyed from location to location. As you read these profiles, it's interesting to note how individual careers evolved during years of service in the Marine Corps. One Marine started out as a cook and became the head drill instructor for the Special Training Company, a prestigious physical fitness assignment. Another saw combat in Vietnam as a corporal and was decorated for valor in combat. He left the Corps and returned later as a chaplain. We even met a British Royal Marine, who was the physical fitness advisor to the commanding officer at OCS in Virginia, a long way from home!

It is our hope that these profiles will provide inspiration to those men and women currently in the Marine Corps or who are considering a future with the Marines. These stories demonstrate that if you are willing and dedicated to advancing your career in the Marines, opportunities abound.

You'll also notice our "fitness in action" close-ups. These are detailed looks at some key fitness programs that are unique to the

Marines. We'll walk you though several training courses, including the confidence course, o'course, circuit course, and stamina course. In many cases these are step-by-step presentations that will provide insight into the techniques and principles behind the events. If you plan on attending recruit training or OCS, you'll appreciate having a mental image beforehand, so you can better prepare yourself for the challenges that lie ahead.

The events may be tough—seemingly impossible at times—but the rewards and benefits you'll gain from looking back and saying to yourself, "Hey, I did that!" are immeasurable. Each vault, each leap, each pull up the rope brings an individual closer and closer to becoming a proud, confident person.

Numerous stories are told of parents who say goodbye to a skinny or overweight son or daughter and who, upon completion

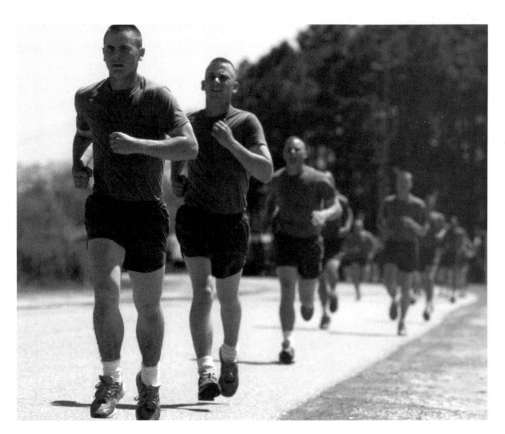

of training, return to barely recognize their child in appearance and demeanor. The weeks of training positively shape both body and spirit.

That's what is unique about the Marine Corps training we witnessed: an awareness of the value of developing a well-rounded Marine. A Marine who is both self-reliant and a team player. A Marine who knows how and when to fight, yet is grounded in moral decency. The Marines build soldiers, but they also shape men and women into responsible citizens.

And throughout, the thread of fitness runs. Taking care of one's health though regular fitness activity is the duty of a Marine. And the Marine Corps promotes fitness as a *lifelong activity*. To that end, the Marines Corps has developed a sophisticated health and wellness program for Marines, their families, and the civilians employed by the Marine Corps. Titled "Semper Fit," this program is composed of nine fundamental elements including physical fitness, nutrition, stress management, and counseling on a variety of important health and mental health subjects.

Semper Fit is a truly progressive vision for the health and wellness of Marines. The mission of Semper Fit is "to incorporate healthy lifestyles into daily living and the challenging work environment by encouraging and promoting wellness and fitness programs, activities, education, and literature for all of its constituents."

From classes on healthy cooking and Yoga, to aerobics and diabetes management, Semper Fit provides a "one stop shop" to Marines looking for a healthier lifestyle.

Our journey with this book took us to many places and introduced us to many great people. More time was spent on this book than any other to date. Every effort was taken with the goal of providing you, the reader, with a book that would give you years of lasting results.

To those men and women of the United States Marine Corps who courageously serve our nation: We thank you! Semper fidelis, Semper fit. Always faithful, always fit! God Bless.

USMC Photo

THE US MARINES: PAST AND PRESENT

Resolved, that two battalions of Marines be raised; that particular care be taken, that no persons be appointed to office, or enlisted into said battalions, but as such are good seamen, or so acquainted with maritime affairs as to be able to serve to advantage by sea when required; that they be enlisted and commissioned to serve for and during the present war between Great Britain and the Colonies, unless dismissed by order of Congress; that they be distinguished by the names of the first and second battalions of American Marines...

Continental Congress, November 10, 1775

On November 10, 1775, in Philadelphia the Continental Congress passed a resolution stating that "two Battalions of Marines be raised" for service as landing forces with the American fleet. This resolution, sponsored by John Adams, established the Continental Marines and marked the birthdate of the United States Marine Corps. Serving on land and at sea, these first Marines distinguished themselves in a number of important operations, including their first amphibious raid into

17

the Bahamas in March 1776, under the command of Captain (later Major) Samuel Nicholas. Nicholas, the first commissioned officer in the Continental Marines, remained the senior Marine officer throughout the American Revolution and is considered to be the first Marine Commandant.

Marines saw action in the quasi-war with France at the turn of the century, landed in Santo Domingo in 1800, and took part in many operations against the Barbary pirates along the "Shores of Tripoli" from 1801 to 1815.

Marines participated in numerous naval operations during the War of 1812. Marines also fought alongside Andrew Jackson in the defeat of the British at New Orleans in 1815. The decades following the War of 1812 saw the Marines protecting American interests around the world, in the Caribbean in 1821 and 1822, at the Falkland Islands in 1832, Sumatra in 1831 to 1832, and off the coast of West Africa from 1820 to 1861, and also close to home in the operations against the Seminole Indians in Florida from 1836 to 1842.

During the Mexican War, Marines seized enemy seaports on both the Gulf and Pacific coasts. While landing parties of Marines and sailors were seizing enemy ports along the coast, a battalion of Marines joined General Scott's army at Puebla and marched and fought all the way to the "Halls of Montezuma," Mexico City.

Marines served ashore and afloat in the Civil War as well (1861-1865). Although most service was with the Navy, a battalion fought at Bull Run and other units saw action with the blockading squadrons and at Cape Hatteras, New Orleans, Charleston, and Fort Fisher. The last third of the nineteenth century saw Marines making numerous landings throughout the world, especially in the Orient and in the Caribbean.

Following the Spanish-American War (1898), in which Marines performed with valor in Cuba, Puerto Rico, Guam, and the Philippines, the Corps en-

Marine Corps Motto:
Semper Fidelis, which means
Always Faithful.

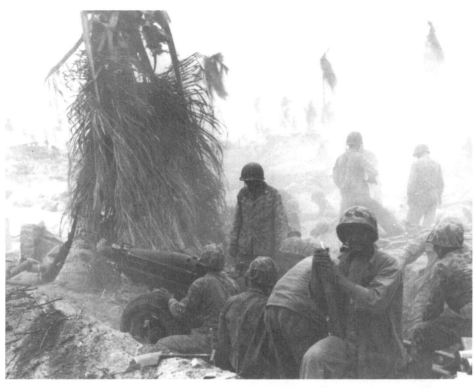

USMC Photo

The Marine standing over the pack howitzer (center) is wearing a helmet with two holes in it. The hole in the side was made as a bullet entered and the one in front as it left. The Marine was wearing the helmet at the time. The smoke is caused by the powder from their own guns and by sand and coral kicked up by projectiles from Japanese guns on Tarawa. 1945

tered an era of expansion and professional development. Marines saw active service in the Philippine Insurrection, the Boxer Rebellion in China, and in numerous other nations, including Nicaragua, Panama, the Dominican Republic, Cuba, Mexico, and Haiti.

In World War I the Marine Corps distinguished itself on the battle-fields of France as the 4th Marine Brigade earned the title of "Devil Dogs" for heroic action at Belleau Wood, Soissons, St. Mihiel, Blanc Mont, and in the final Meuse-Argonne offensive. Marines are still called Devil Dogs in honor of their brave sacrifices in WWI. Marine aviation also played a part in the war effort, flying day bomber missions over France and Belgium. More than 30,000 Marines served in France and more than a third were killed or wounded in six months of intense fighting.

During the two decades before World War II, the Marine Corps began to develop in earnest the doctrine, equipment, and organization needed for amphibious warfare. The success of this effort was proven in many battles during World War II. By the end of the war in 1945, the Marine Corps had grown to include six divisions, five air wings, and supporting troops. Its strength in World War II peaked at 485,113, though the Marines paid a heavy cost in terms of number of troops dead or injured. Nearly 87,000 were either dead and

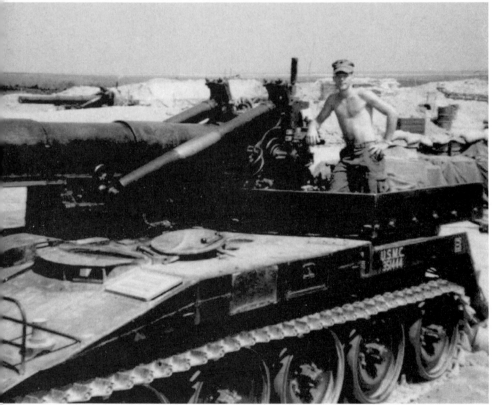

Combat operations just south of Con Thien, Vietnam, 1968. Bravo Platoon, 1st 8" Howitzer Battery (SP), supported Marine operations throughout Leatherneck Square with deadly accuracy.

Thomas F. Sullivan, Jr

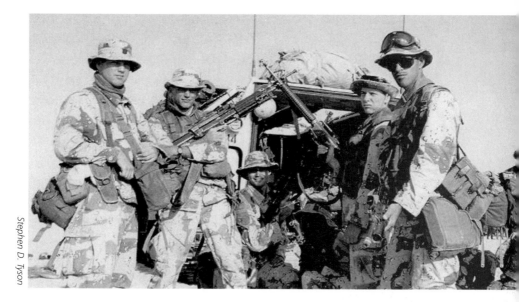

Stephen D. Tyson

Operation Desert Storm, 1991. Marines take a break from Gulf War action.

wounded at the end of World War II, and 81 Marines had earned the Medal of Honor.

The landing of the 9th Marine Expeditionary Brigade at Da Nang in 1965 marked the beginning of large-scale Marine involvement in Vietnam. By summer 1968, after the enemy's Tet Offensive, Marine Corps strength in Vietnam rose to a peak of approximately 85,000. The Vietnam War, the longest in the history of the Marine Corps, exacted a high cost as well with over 13,000 Marines killed and more than 88,000 wounded.

In the mid-1970s, the Marine Corps played a key role in the development of the Rapid Deployment Force, a multi-service organization created to insure a flexible, timely military response around the world when needed. The Maritime Prepositioning Ships (MPS) concept was developed to enhance this capability by pre-staging equipment needed for combat in the vicinity of the designated area of operations, and reduce response time as Marines traveled by air to linkup with MPS assets.

Overshadowed by the events in the Persian Gulf during 1990-91,

"Among the men who fought on Iwo Jima, Uncommon Valor was a common virtue."

—Admiral Chester W. Nimitz, 1945

during which the 1st and 2d Marine Divisions breached the Iraqi defense lines and stormed into occupied Kuwait and two Marine Expeditionary Brigades held in check some 50,000 Iraqis along the Kuwait coast, were a number of other significant Marine deployments demonstrating the Corps' flexible and rapid response. Some of these missions included many non-combatant evacuation operations, such as the rescuing of civilians and diplomats in Liberia and Somalia, and humanitarian lifesaving operations in Bangladesh, the Philippines, and northern Iraq.

Marines are also often actively engaged in providing assistance to the nation's counter-drug effort, assisting in battling wild fires in the western United States, and aiding in flood and hurricane relief operations.

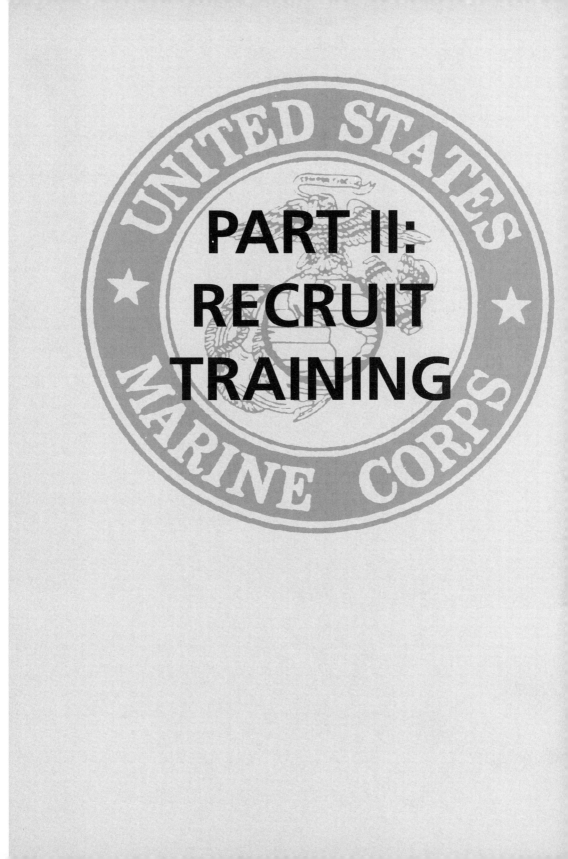

PART II: RECRUIT TRAINING

WELCOME TO USMC BOOTCAMP!

AN OVERVIEW

Upon their arrival at Boot Camp, each recruit is met by a Drill Instructor (D.I.). Experienced in training recruits to perform as a team, DIs supervise recruits' performance in all facets of training and evaluate their progress. A platoon normally consists of a Senior Drill Instructor and two to three Assistant Drill Instructors. The responsibility of the Senior Drill Instructor is to ensure that each recruit is given ample opportunity to complete each portion of training and to handle any problems a recruit may have.

Recruit training is conducted at either of the two Marine Corps Recruit Depots (MCRDs): Parris Island, South Carolina or San Diego, California, depending upon where the recruit resides. All female recruits train at Parris Island.

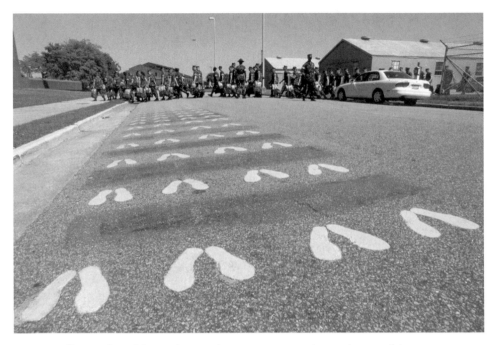

Yellow painted footprints welcome new recruits at the receiving area. Recruits are ordered off the bus and onto the footprints. While standing at attention, these new recruits will receive their first instructions from the Drill Instructor.

PROCESSING AND FORMING

Immediately upon arrival at recruit training, recruits are assigned to a platoon. For males there are six to eight platoons of 50-88 recruits and for females there are two platoons of 45-55 recruits that begin training at the same time. Each platoon is assigned a living area (squad bay), and each recruit is assigned a rack (bed) and storage locker.

Recruits spend up to seven days in processing and forming. Their first day begins very early in the morning with reveille, breakfast, haircuts (males only), showers, and the issuing of personal gear items.

During the following days recruits are given a medical and dental examination, store their civilian clothing, undergo administrative processing, and take a battery of aptitude tests. They also take an Initial Strength Test (IST). Recruits must pass the IST to start training. Recruits who fail to achieve the minimum standards are sent to the Physical Conditioning Platoon for remedial training.

INITIAL STRENGTH TEST (MINIMUM STANDARDS)

Males	
Pull-ups	2
Situps	35 in two minutes
1.5 Mile Run	13 minutes :30 seconds

Females	
Flex-Arm Hang	17 seconds
Situps	35 in two minutes
1 Mile Run	10 minutes :30 seconds

Also during processing and forming, recruits receive instruction on basic drill movements, customs and courtesies, rank structure, barracks procedures and personal hygiene. These future Marines are also issued a rifle. At the end of processing and forming they are ready to start their training.

TRAINING DAYS

During their first few weeks of training, recruits learn how to make their rack, keep their squad bay clean, wear their uniform correctly, conduct close order drill, and participate in physical training (PT). Recruits learn how to act and react as a team. They attend classes, take tests, run the obstacle course, learn combat water survival techniques and more.

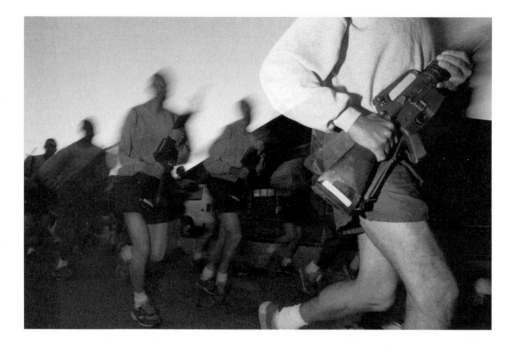

Recruits go to the rifle range where they will learn safety, maintenance of their weapon, and, of course, accurate shooting. Naturally, this is some of the most important training recruits receive. Recruits must qualify on the rifle range to progress to the next level of training.

Physical training becomes more challenging as training continues. Recruits undergo Basic Warrior Training (BWT) and Tactical Weapons Firing. They learn everything from fast roping to night firing of weapons. They are taught to fire a variety of light infantry weapons, and learn basic field skills such as land navigation; Nuclear, Biological, Chemical (NBC) warfare; and rappelling.

THE CRUCIBLE

The defining moment of every Marine's recruit training comes during the Crucible—a test that demands every ounce of physical and mental strength a recruit can muster. Every recruit must pass this awesome test in order to become a Marine. The Crucible is a 54 hour challenge consisting of: a day movement resupply, a casualty evacuation, a combat assault course, a reaction course, an unknown distance firing course, a night infiltration course, and a night march. The events are designed to emphasize teamwork, self-confidence, and core values.

The Crucible ends with a Colors ceremony, followed by the Drill Instructors distributing the Marine Corps eagle, globe and anchor to each of their recruits, signifying that these men and women have successfully advanced into the Marine Corps.

Graduation follows soon afterward. For all their hard work and determination, recruits earn the title "United States Marine."

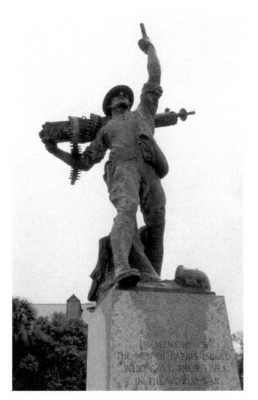

Dedicated in 1924 to the memory of those Marines who gave their lives during WWI, this statue is nicknamed "Iron Mike."

"Freedom has a flavor the protected never know."

—*Anonymous Marine,*
Khe Sahn, 1968

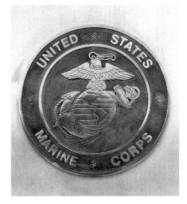

The Marine Corps "Eagle, Globe and Anchor." The Eagle symbolizes the Nation, the Globe signifies World Wide Service, and the Anchor represents Naval Tradition.

RECRUIT
PHYSICAL TRAINING

The ultimate weapon of a Marine is him or herself, and keeping their self healthy is a good behavior that is desired by the Marine Corps. Physical conditioning is one of those things that's part of keeping healthy.

–Tim Bockelman, Physical
Fitness Advisor, Parris Island

Just 64 training days to make a Marine. That's all. And of those 64 days, 64 and 1/2 hours are dedicated exclusively to physical training. The goal: to develop within each Marine recruit a commitment to building and maintaining their level of physical fitness while preparing them for the demanding requirements of Marine Corps life.

The yardstick by which these Marine recruits are measured is the Marine Corps Physical Fitness Test (PFT). The physical fitness conditioning level of each recruit is tested on Day 40 of the training cycle. Three events comprise the PFT: pull-ups (or flex-arm hangs for women), situps, and a run.

MARINE CORPS PFT

Males	Minimum	Maximum
Pull-ups	3	20
Situps	40 in two minutes	80 in two minutes
3 Mile Run	28 minutes	18 minutes or less

Females	Minimum	Maximum
Flex-Arm Hang	23 seconds	70 seconds
Situps	40 in two minutes	80 in two minutes
3 Mile Run	31 minutes	21 minutes or less

Recruit physical training consists of a variety of fitness challenges including: running, circuit courses, calisthenics, strength condition-

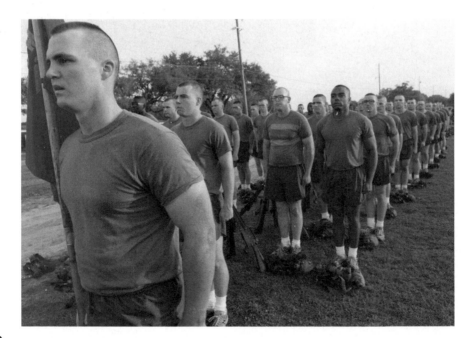

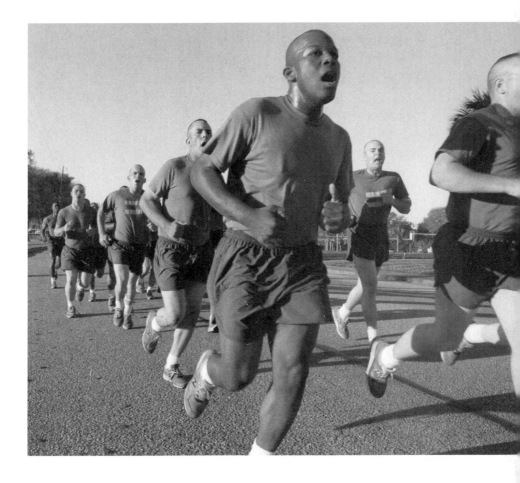

ing, and the obstacle course. A Marine learns to use his or her own body weight for resistance during exercises, so that wherever a Marine goes, he or she can stay fit in a variety of ways.

Runs are conducted in a number of ways. A **FORMATION RUN** has the recruit training company following the same pace. On Training Day 1, the distance is one and a half miles and the pace is a nine minute mile. By Training Day 43, Formation Runs are up to three miles in distance.

SQUAD ABILITY RUNS group the recruits by their running capacity: fast, average, and slow. The Drill Instructor sets the pace for each running squad. Often, interval training is utilized during these runs to increase overall performance.

INDIVIDUAL EFFORT RUNS are "personal best" efforts. Each recruit is allowed to run at their own pace.

TABLE EXERCISES are a common PT activity during recruit training. These are a series of conditioning calisthenics and dynamic exercises which work all muscle groups. Pushups, crunches, and side straddle hops are just a few examples.

STRENGTH CONDITIONING exercises include pull-ups, dips, pushups, hanging knee raises, and rope climbing. A combination of these exercises is found on the circuit course, an exciting fitness challenge which is highlighted in this book.

Another exercise event is **RIFLE PT**. Recruits learn to use their M-16 as a resistance source as effectively as free weights. Weighing in at 8.6 pounds with the clip removed, you may not think it's a lot of weight, but once you've completed 200 repetitions in a combination of moves, you'll reconsider!

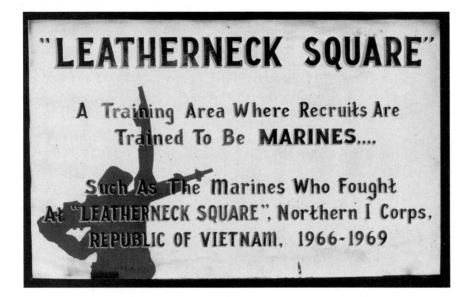

"LEATHERNECK SQUARE"

A Training Area Where Recruits Are Trained To Be **MARINES**....

Such As The Marines Who Fought At "LEATHERNECK SQUARE", Northern I Corps, REPUBLIC OF VIETNAM, 1966-1969

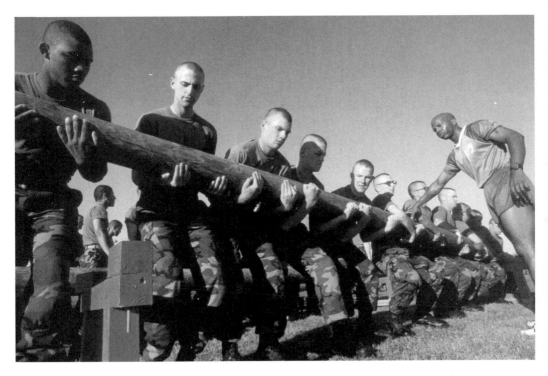

Rifle PT exercises work a variety of different muscle groups. The exercises include: *the foreup behind the back*, much like a military shoulder press; *the lunge side turn and bend*, which works the abdominal and lower leg muscle groups; *the foreup back bend*, which stretches the abdominals; and *the up and forward*, which strengthens the shoulder muscles, the deltoids.

LOG DRILLS are another fitness activity. Although there is a strength component to Log Drills, in recruit training these drills are used primarily as a teamwork-building activity.

A single recruit can't lift that log by himself. But when eight to twelve people work together they're able to put it over their head safely. With this activity, the Marine Corps is working on team skills—the ability to work together—a vital component of Marine Corps life.

NICKNAMES OF LOGS:
Humongous One, Gargantuan, Sweet Caroline, Wild Thing, John Wayne, Chesty, Gung Ho, The Beast, Dan Daly

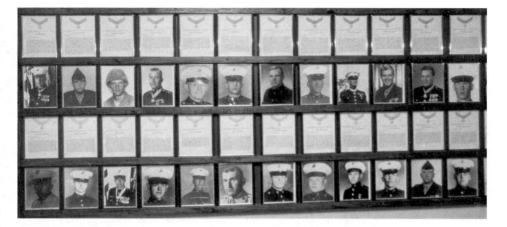

For recruits assigned to the Special Training Company, The Medal of Honor Wall serves as a vivid reminder that physical adversity comes with the job of being a Marine.

THE SPECIAL TRAINING COMPANY

The Special Training Company has two functions: to rehabilitate those recruits who are injured in training and to physically condition those recruits who are not in proper condition to start recruit training or who are unable to keep up with the rigorous physical training regimen.

The 5% or so of recruits who do not pass the initial strength test are assigned to the **Physical Conditioning Platoon**, which lasts three weeks for the males and two weeks for the females. After their stay in the physical conditioning platoon, these recruits will take the Initial Strength Test again and begin regular recruit training. In essence, the physical conditioning platoon acts as a "pre-training phase" for those recruits who are unable to meet the initial physical fitness requirements. The goal is to get these recruits "up to speed."

Females are on a two-week cycle because their problems are usu-

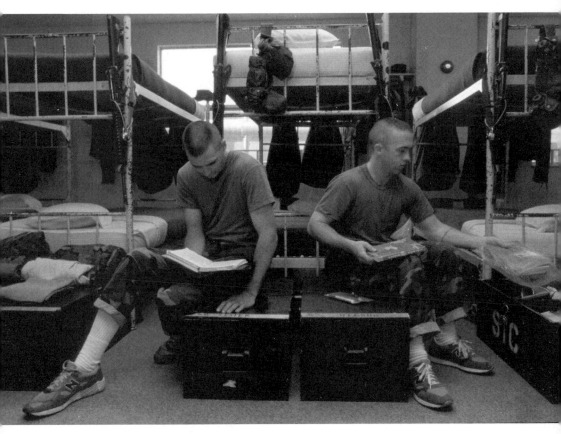

Down time in the Special Training Company barracks.

ally situps or running, two areas where recruits seem to improve more quickly. The two-week pre-training schedule fits in well because every two weeks a new female series begins. For the males, the harder issue is pull-ups.

There are hard training days three times a week, usually Monday, Wednesday and Friday, which include some outdoor training followed by the Daily 16. In the afternoon recruits will also go to the gym, where they'll work on general conditioning as well as targeting their specific conditioning needs. Tuesdays and Thursdays are lighter workout days, allowing for recovery. *It is important to allow your body time to recover from working out. This is where the fitness benefits take hold!*

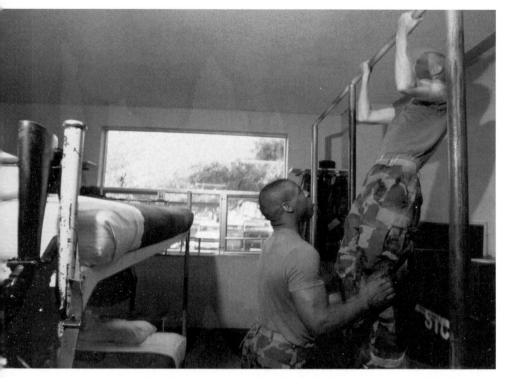

Recruits practice chin-ups in the Special Training Company barracks.

Most recruits in the Physical Conditioning Platoon make it through the pre-training on schedule.

The Medical Rehabilitation Platoon provides medical supervision, physical rehabilitation, and limited training for recruits who have been found to be temporarily unable to participate in normal training due to medical problems, while also providing the necessary guidance to maintain motivation to return to training.

TIMOTHY L. BOCKELMAN

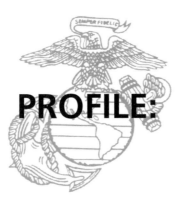

PROFILE:

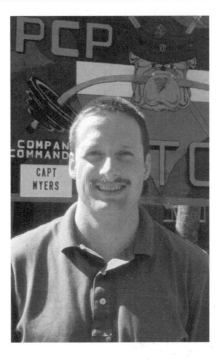

Originally from Fostoria, Ohio, Tim Bockelman graduated from the University of Toledo with a degree in Physical Education and Kinesiotherapy. Tim has served as the Fitness Counselor for Owen-Illinois, Inc., as well as the Staff Kinesiotherapist at the University of Toledo. In 1987, Tim was promoted to Program Coordinator for Occupational Ergogenics (Work Hardening) at the University.

In 1989, Tim was hired by the Marine Corps as a Physical Fitness Advisor. This position established Tim as the Depot's only professional fitness expert, charged with providing recommendations to commanders at all levels concerning fitness issues.

Tim currently resides in South Carolina with his wife and two children. He continues to lead Marine Corps recruits as their Fitness Advisor, developing fitness programs for the Marines.

CLOSE-UP: CIRCUIT COURSE

A circuit course is made up of a series of exercise stations arranged to develop strength and endurance. A circuit course can be set up indoors or outdoors, and is relatively simple. A large number of Marines can be trained simultaneously on a circuit course. Whether you want to be a Marine, or just train like one, you can improve these exercises at your gym or in your backyard with minimal investment.

The circuit course is comprised of ten exercise stations. At each station the specified exercise is repeated for 60 seconds. When the D.I.'s whistle is blown, recruits shift to the next station. Recruits have 60 seconds to move to the next station and begin exercising. This 60 seconds "on station"/60 seconds "change stations" drill is conducted until everyone has rotated through the stations on the circuit course.

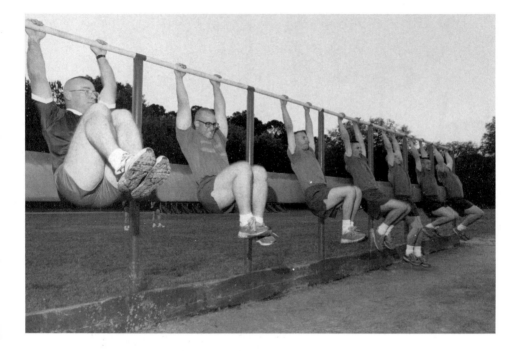

HANGING KNEE RAISES

Grab the bar above your head and lift your knees up to the height of your hips. Now reverse the motion. And repeat. This exercise works the hip flexors.

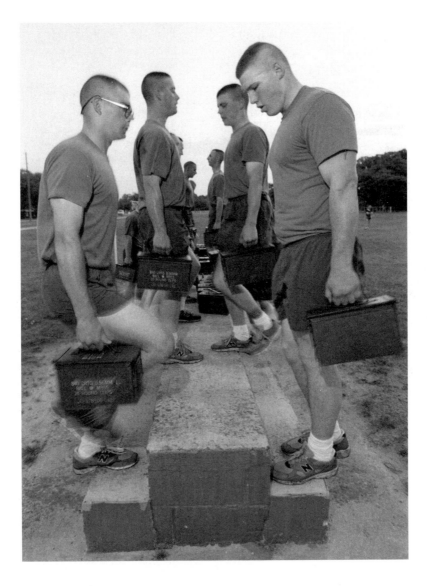

STEP-UPS WITH AMMO BOXES

Not your typical aerobic step-class! This time you're hanging on to ammo boxes filled with 25 pounds of cement. Or you can choose dumbbells. Either way, you're giving your thigh muscles (quadriceps) a great cardio workout!

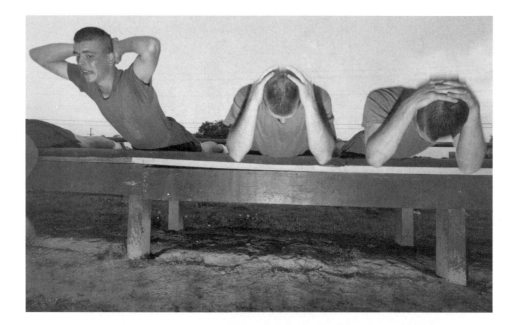

BACK EXTENSIONS

Here's how we strengthen your lower back. Lay on the platform with your torso held in front of the platform and your legs hooked under the bar for security. Gently raise and lower your torso, being careful not to hyperextend your back when you come up.

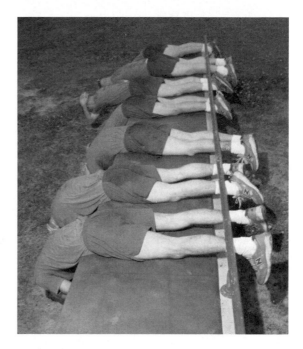

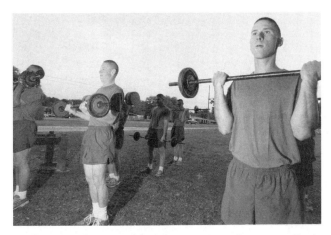

BICEPS CURLS

Use a standard curl bar of about 35-40 pounds (or make one from pipe, coffee cans, and cement) and raise and lower the weight using a smooth, controlled motion. Concentrate on keeping the exercise in your biceps. Bend your knees slightly and don't use your lower back to perform the repetitions!

PUSHUPS

Be a Marine and do them right and tight! Eyes ahead, back straight and it's up and down. Work your chest and those shoulders!

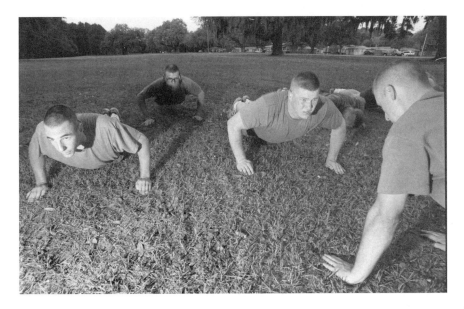

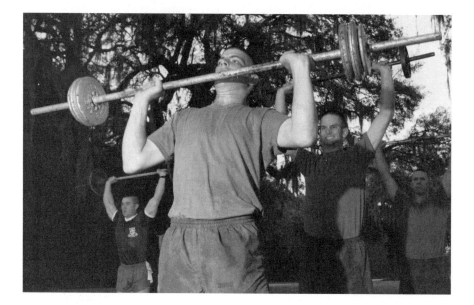

MILITARY PRESS

Using a standard curl bar again (or your homemade version) load up with anywhere from 20-50 lbs. Keep your knees bent and spread your leg ahead and behind you to create a stable position. Again, protect your back to avoid injury. Shoulders are the target this time.

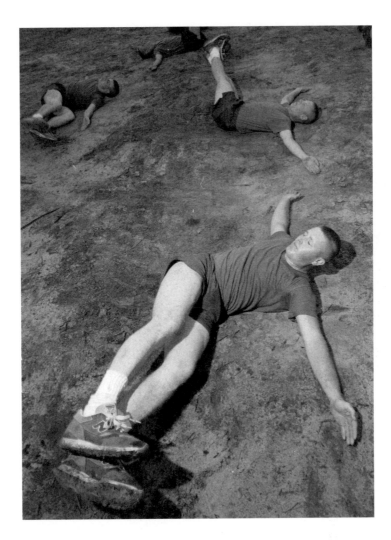

BODY TWISTS

Give your upper body a rest for a few as you focus on your mid-section, also known as the abdominals. This exercise works the side abdominals (obliques) and is performed as follows: lie on your back as shown. Lift your legs to a 90 degree angle to your torso. Swing your legs from side to side in a controlled motion as you feel the heat in your obliques!

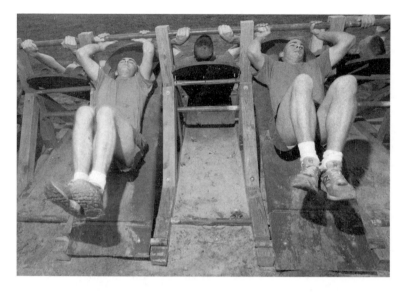

INCLINED SITUPS

This exercise is performed on a slanted bench. Lay on your back with your head uphill. Raise and lower your knees to your chest so your hips leave the bench. This exercise works the lower abdominal muscles.

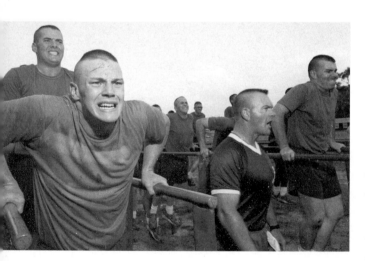

DIPS

This exercise works the triceps. When doing them, make certain not to dip too low. Remember to raise and lower yourself in a controlled motion. Don't bend your elbows beyond 90 degrees.

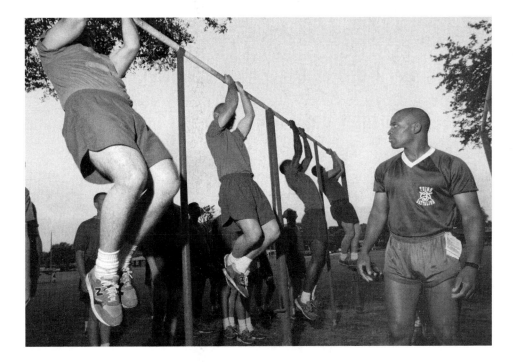

CHIN-UPS

Marines love to do chin-ups! They are an excellent way to build your strength, especially in your back and shoulders. With your hands about shoulder width apart, palms facing toward you, grab the bar and pull yourself up. Do it in a smooth motion. Look skyward as you pull up. This will help concentrate the exercise on the proper muscle groups.

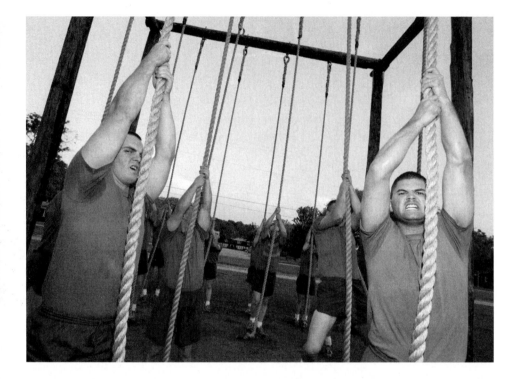

ROPE HEAVES

Another upper body strengthener. Forearm, biceps, and chest—all get worked as you grip the rope with your hands while your feet are free. Lift yourself up and down keeping your grip tight on the rope. Don't start climbing! Stay in the same place while you repeat the motion for the duration of the 60 second cycle.

CLOSE-UP: THE USMC RECRUIT OBSTACLE COURSE

Every branch of the military includes an obstacle course as a component of both recruit and officer training, and the Marines are no exception. Each training company is provided with its own obstacle course, designed to build strength, speed, confidence, and coordination. During basic training, Marine recruits are required to complete four hours of instruction on the obstacle course.

> "No one can say that the Marines have ever failed to do their work in handsome fashion."
>
> —Major General Johnson Hagood, U.S. Army

The Marine Corps obstacle course is a classic, run in a straight line from start to finish. Most of the obstacles require vaulting skills, and a few require brute strength, but all of the obstacles demand proper technique and a willingness to overcome fear. Although there is no time requirement for completing the obstacle course, most recruits accomplish the task in less than three minutes. We'll take a look at each obstacle, and the skills it requires.

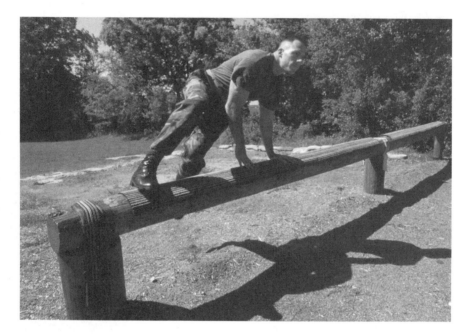

LOW HURDLE

Up and over. Not so bad! Then again, it's early.

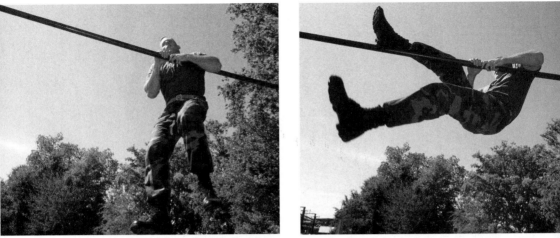

These photos demonstrate the chicken wing method.

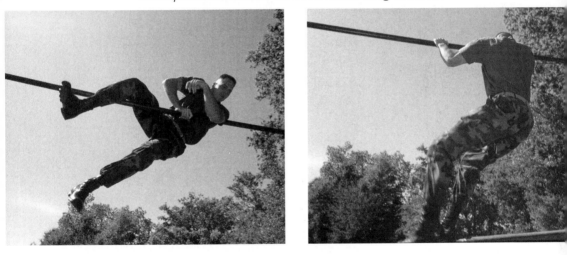

SINGLE HIGH BAR

This is the first big obstacle, and there are two ways to negotiate it. One is called the chicken wing method, where you jump up and grab the bar underneath, then throw your legs up and roll yourself over the top of the bar. Another way is the kicking method in which you use a kick similar to one used in gymnastics and swing yourself under and over the bar.

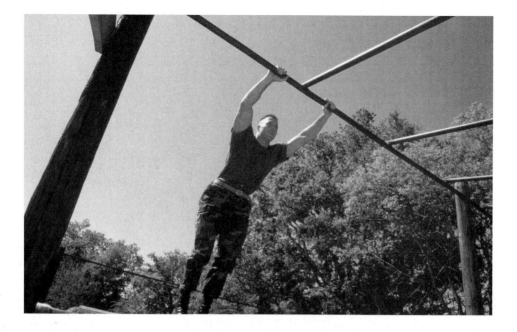

COMBINATION: SLANTED BAR/BALANCE LOG

Grab the bars, swing your legs up, and shimmy down the bar hand under hand and hanging upside down. Then you'll traverse a balance log that angles downward, much like a

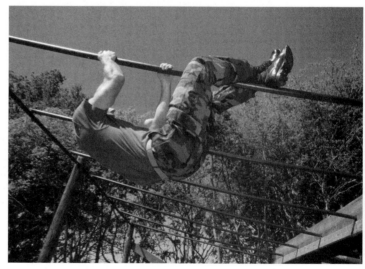

balance beam. The height of the log at the start is seven feet, and it slopes down to about four feet from the ground. Moving quickly is the best way to keep your balance.

At the end of this log you'll meet another log. Jump off and hit it square in your belly. Swing yourself over the top and drop to the ground. It's a seven-foot drop into the soft sawdust.

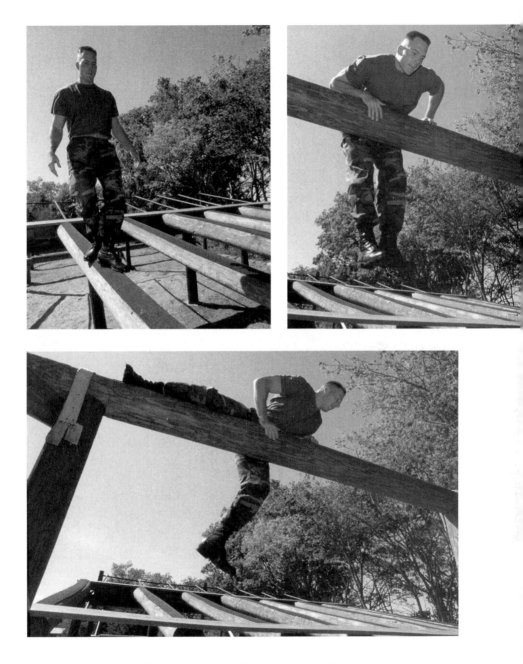

Why sawdust? The sawdust will absorb the shock when you are landing. Bend your knees when you land and grab some sawdust!

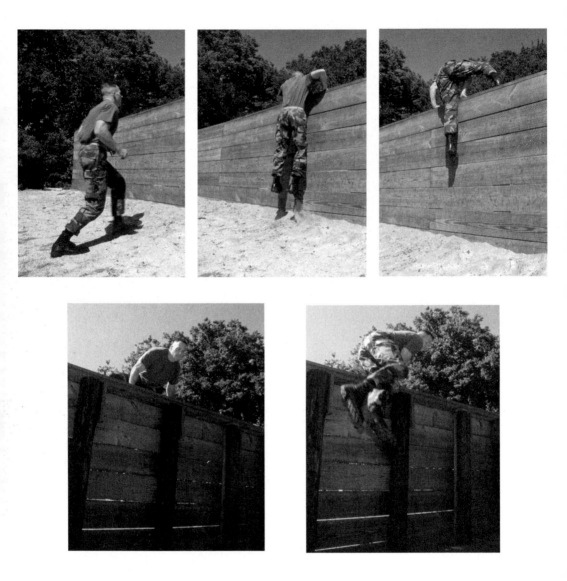

WALL

Hit the wall running. At six feet high, this obstacle is a challenge for most. Use your abdominal muscles and a little coordination to sweep your legs up and over the wall.

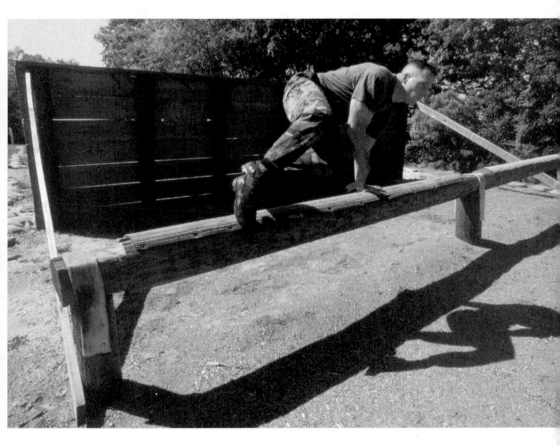

SINGLE HURDLE

Easy one. Catch your breath. You're going to need it!

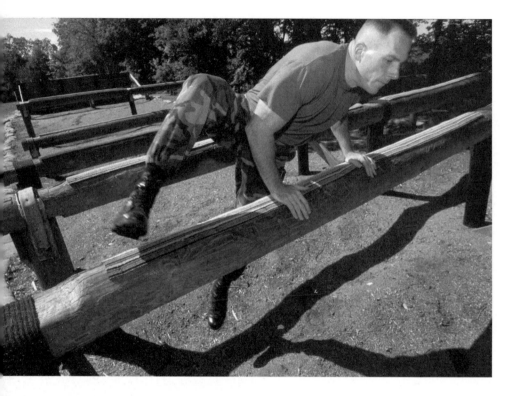

MULTIPLE HURDLE

Four chest-high hurdles await. There are a couple of different tech-niques to get this one successfully accomplished. You might lay your body on it, swinging your legs over and pushing off as seen in the photo. Or you might do a hand hurdle, much like a gymnastics vault.

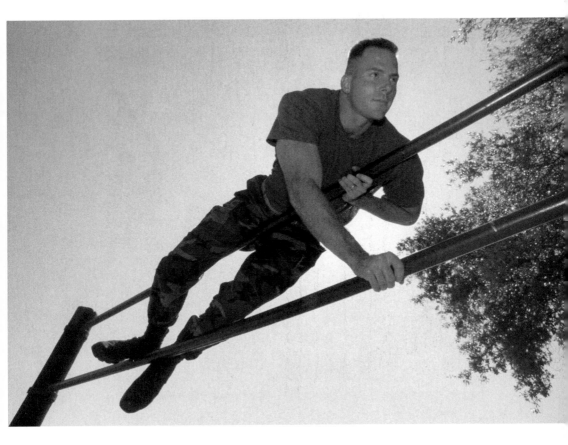

DOUBLE HIGH BAR

The next obstacle is a double high bar. The goal is to go over the top bar, which by itself is probably too high to negotiate. But there is a lower bar there to make it easier. Climb up onto the lower bar, using the chicken wing method. Bring a leg up onto the lower bar, and swing your other leg up to the top bar, at the same time grabbing the top bar. Then crawl over the top bar, pushing away as you're jumping down. Bend those knees and grab some more sawdust when you land!

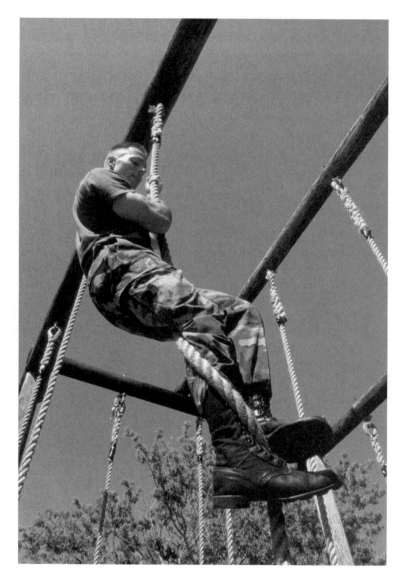

ROPE CLIMB

There are a couple of different techniques for climbing rope, but usually the most common technique is the brake-and-squat technique. This method uses your leg and abdominal muscles to do most of the work, rather than just using your arms.

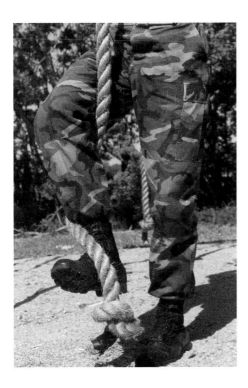 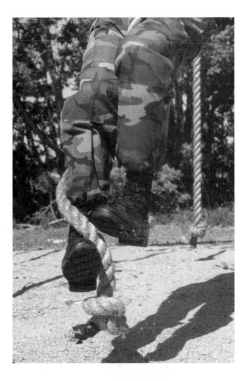

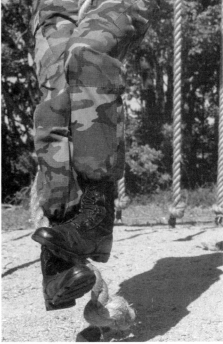

Proper technique for wrapping the rope around your legs is seen in the photos. The friction between your boots and the rope will keep you from slipping downward as you progress up the rope.

CLOSE-UP: COMBAT WATER SURVIVAL TRAINING

Author's note: *We have included this section to show the broad scope of Marine recruit training. Although not considered a part of fitness training per se, it is an important component in the overall physical readiness of a Marine. Please consult with a local swim club or contact the American Red Cross for proper swimming and water safety instruction. Swimming is a highly dangerous activity. Do not attempt these drills without proper instruction, supervision, and safety precautions.*

The inherent nature of Marine Corps operations and training requires that Marines have the ability to survive in water. Combat water survival training is designed to reduce fear of water, instill self-confidence, and develop the individual Marine's ability to survive in water.

Combat Water Survival is physically and mentally demanding, especially for some of the recruits that are not very strong or confident around water.

The minimum qualification level for all enlisted Marines is Combat Water Survival, Fourth Class (CWS4). Entry level CWS training is con-

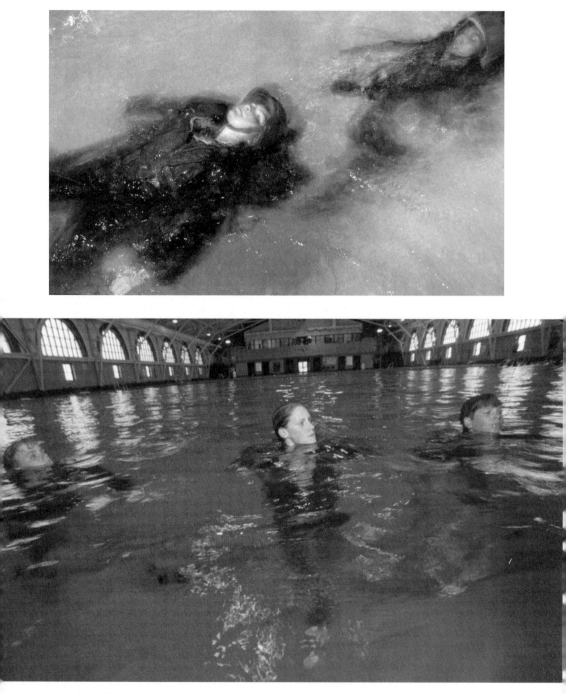

Qualifying for Combat Water Survival Fourth Class (CWS4).

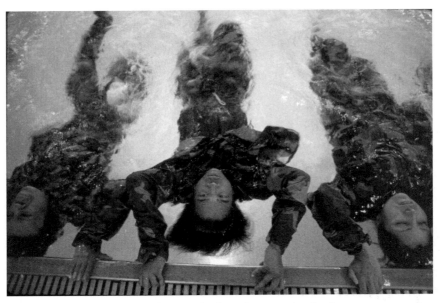

Recruits increase their confidence by learning to relax in the water.

ducted at both the San Diego and Parris Island recruit depots. Emphasis is on personal survival without gear. CSW4 includes instruction on the Beginner Swimmer Stroke (front and back), drown-proofing, and treading water.

The qualifications for CWS4 are as follows (uniform is blouse and trousers only, without boots).

- Enter shallow water (minimum one meter in depth). Swim 25 meters in shallow water using either the Beginners Swimmer Stroke (front or back), or any other survival stroke.

- Step into deep water from a minimum height of eight feet and a maximum of 15 feet using the abandon ship technique. Tread water for 2 minutes, then drown-proof for 2 minutes face down.

- Without exiting the water, inflate blouse and float for 1 minute, then deflate blouse and swim for 25 meters.

Many recruits advance beyond the basic requirement of CSW4 and aim for Combat Water Survival Third Class (CWS3) during their recruit

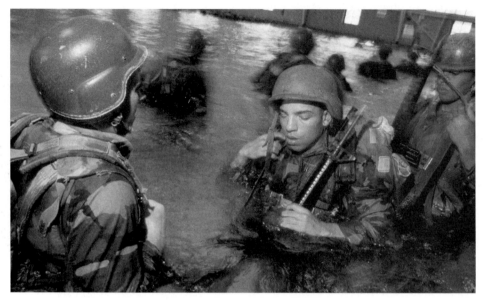

Marine recruits qualify for CWS 3.

training. The emphasis of CSW3 is on personal survival under combat situations and while on maneuvers.

The qualifications for CWS3 are as follows (uniform is full combat gear, including boots).

- Enter shallow water (minimum one meter in depth) with rubberized training rifle and wearing full combat gear (pack and helmet), walk 20 meters in waist deep water with rifle held in front.

- Walk 40 meters in chest deep water wearing full combat gear and with rifle slung around neck. Use a modified breast stroke arm movement and modified combat stroke (bicycle stroke) kick.

- Swim for 40 meters in deep water (over the head) with full combat gear and rifle.

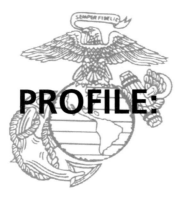

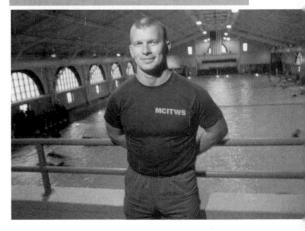

PROFILE:

Originally from Hazelton, Pennsylvania, Staff Sergeant Simpson joined the Marine Corps in 1985 at Parris Island, South Carolina. Upon completing his first tour in South Carolina, Staff Sergeant Simpson continued his training by attending Airborne, Ranger and Water Survival Swim Instructor Schools.

In early 1989, Simpson transferred to Hawaii, where he was stationed at Kaneohe Bay. He was the Water Survival Swim School instructor there and later became an open water Life Guard and rescue swimmer. Simpson then moved to Pearl Harbor where he was assigned as the Platoon Sergeant of a reactionary force to guard the decommissioning of several nuclear submarines.

In 1991, Simpson traveled to Cuba to provide fence line security, becoming the Platoon Sergeant for the reaction team during the Haitian Crisis. In 1992 he returned to Parris Island where he became a Drill Instructor. While in this position, he traveled to Quantico, Virginia to become an Instructor Trainer of Water Survival. He then spent two years at Parris Island training recruits in water survival qualification.

In 1995, Simpson sailed aboard USS THEODORE ROOSEVELT and deployed to the Mediterranean during the Bosnia conflict. He then reported back to Parris Island and was put in charge of the Combat Training Pool.

Currently, Staff Sergeant Simpson remains the Combat Training Pool Director at Parris Island, is a certified Emergency Medical Technician, and continues to train and compete in athletic events throughout the year. Most recently he was selected from among 1400 applicants to participate in one of the world's toughest athletic challenges, The Eco-Challenge, a 350-mile endurance race, to take place in Morocco later this year.

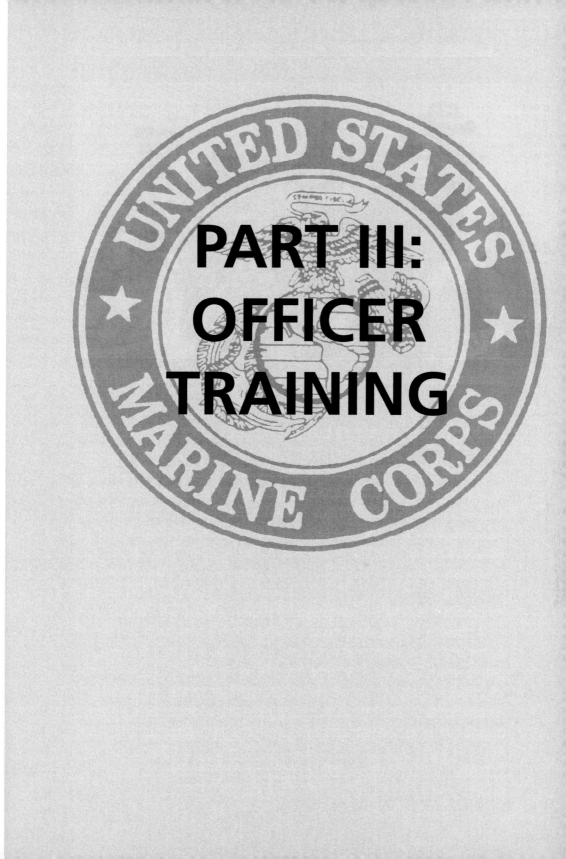

PART III:
OFFICER
TRAINING

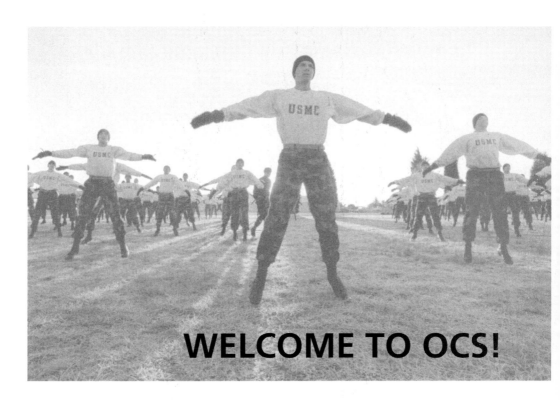

WELCOME TO OCS!

The mission of Officer Candidates School (OCS) is to train, evaluate, and screen officer candidates to ensure that they possess the moral, intellectual, and physical qualities for commissioning and the leadership potential to serve successfully as officers in the United States Marines.

The approach in training officers is fundamentally different than the approach used to train recruits. The end product of recruit training is a basic Marine that will obey, react, and follow orders under the stress of combat.

The end product of OCS is a Lieutenant who has exhibited the potential to think and lead under the stress of combat. Above all else, future Marine officers must be leaders. A key method of determining a candidate's leadership potential is their ability to think and function under conditions of chaos and uncertainty.

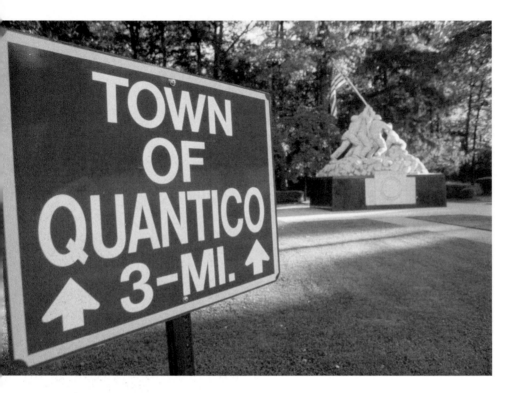

OCS TRAINING PHASES

In-Processing Phase: This first phase is a low stress environment and begins when a candidate arrives at OCS and ends when administrative and medical screenings are complete. This phase is approximately three to five days long.

Transition Training Phase: The second phase begins with the formation of the training company and introduction of the company commander and lasts about two weeks. Training is intensive with emphasis placed on discipline, OCS procedures, and teamwork. This phase also presents the basic instruction necessary for the evaluations conducted during the third phase.

Evaluation Phase: Tests, graded events, graded practical application, and constant and thorough observation by the staff characterize the evaluation phase. Special emphasis is placed on self-discipline and teamwork. Candidates are closely evaluated to determine if they possess the qualities necessary for commissioning.

Out-Processing Phase: This final phase begins following the last graded event and ends on graduation day. The week long phase focuses on the transition to The Basic School (TBS) and final preparation for graduation and commissioning. At TBS, the real officer training begins.

THE OCS CRUCIBLE

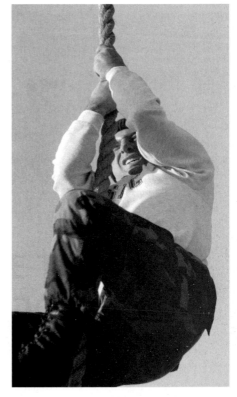

All training conducted at OCS has as its primary purpose to provide a vehicle by which candidates can be evaluated. Although each candidate is graded on their individual performance as a squad or fire team leader, the events are all executed as teams with candidates reverting from leader to team member as the exercises progress. Team members must count on one another in order to successfully complete the task at hand. The capstone exercise, the "OCS Crucible," is the final practical application by which the candidates are tested for their leadership, teamwork, tactics, endurance, and core values assimilation.

"The Marines have never shone more brightly that this morning."

—General Douglas MacArthur, 1950

The OCS Crucible is a three-day long experience. Awakening at midnight, the OCS Crucible starts with a nine-mile night hike, followed by a day of tactical challenges which must be overcome by

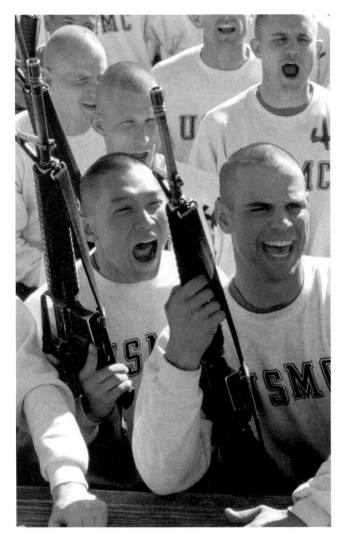

the squad. Sleep comes at midnight, twenty four hours after the first reveille.

The second day begins in the early morning darkness. More squad management problems, including squad resupply and squad movement, must be overcome throughout the long day. The second night candidates conduct squad-sized infiltration exercises, testing their land navigation and leadership skills. By the end of the second night, each candidate will have force marched over 24 miles and participated in 13 to 15 squad attacks in a 48-hour period—all on less than six hours of sleep and four meals.

The final day begins with a helicopter movement to The Basic School (TBS) where candidates, under the leadership of a TBS Lieutenant student, will negotiate a 3-mile run and face the NATO obstacle course. The day ends with lieutenants and candidates eating a meal together and discussing future challenges as Marines. This day represents the bridge between candidate and lieutenant.

Although the "OCS Crucible" is a cumulative test of a candidate's physical, intellectual, and moral fiber while at OCS, most are well prepared for the challenge.

OCS PHYSICAL TRAINING

The intensity of OCS physical training is fantastic. Officer candidates are required to complete 120 hours of physical training including daily Table Exercises, rope climbs, the Obstacle Course, the Confidence Course, the Tarzan Course, the Stamina Course, the Endurance Course, and plenty of running and force marches, more positively referred to as "conditioning hikes."

To be an Officer in the United States Marine Corps you must lead by example. You must keep going when others would quit. You must develop deep reserves of mental and physical strength, ready to be tapped at moment's notice. It is evident that the physical challenges faced at OCS are adequately preparing these men and women for the day when they will be Marine Corps leaders.

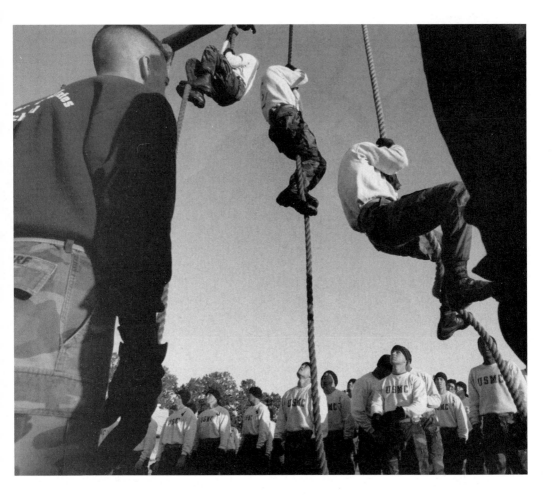

The **Upper Body Development (UBD) Course** is a physical training event typical of the OCS challenge. The UBD Course is a circuit type course which is designed to improve upper body strength and endurance through a series of exercises: rope heaves, inclined pushups, fireman's carry, biceps curls, crunches, long jumps, pull-ups, triceps dips, dorsal raises, and situps. Each station is worked for a specified number of repetitions according to the level of intensity.

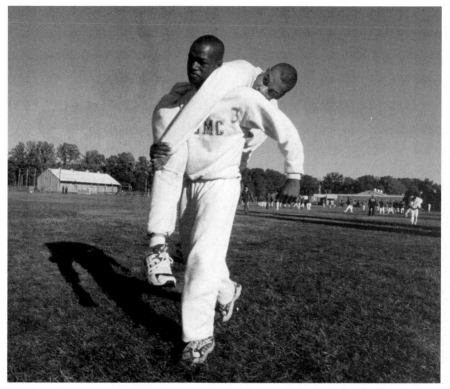

Fireman's carry. OCS UBD Course.

Situps. OCS UBD Course.

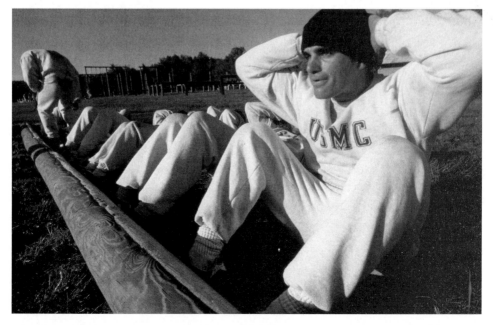

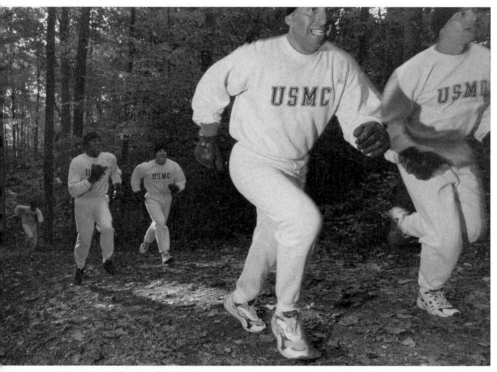

Sprinting the Fartlek Course.

The **Fartlek Course** is another training event which combines running and calisthenics. The Fartlek Course is designed to develop strength, stamina, and endurance—the fundamentals of military fitness. The course consists of a trail run with intermittent exercise stations along the way. Officer Candidates run the trail in squad formation. When they arrive at an exercise station, they perform the specified number of repetitions and continue down the trail to the next station.

Station exercises found along the Fartlek Course include situps, pushups, squat thrusts, sprints, pull-ups, and mountain climbers, which are performed like a double time in place, only with your hands on the ground.

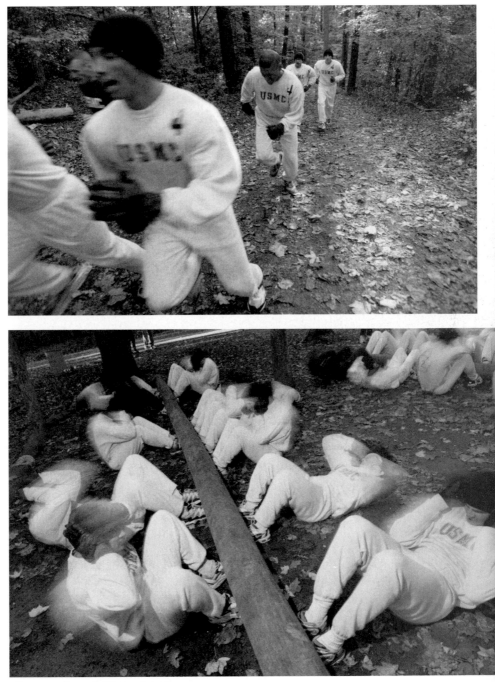

Situp station. OCS Fartlek Course.

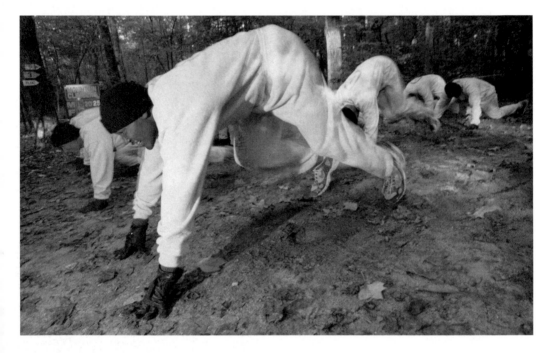

Mountain climbers. OCS Fartlek Course.

At Marine Corps OCS passing the PFT is a given. The goal of training is to develop a lifelong commitment to physical fitness and to gain the knowledge to care for the well-being of your troops. The physical fitness of any military unit is a precious asset. Marine Corps Officers know this. Officer Candidates learn it. Every day.

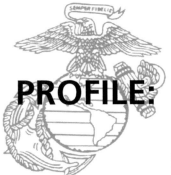

PROFILE:

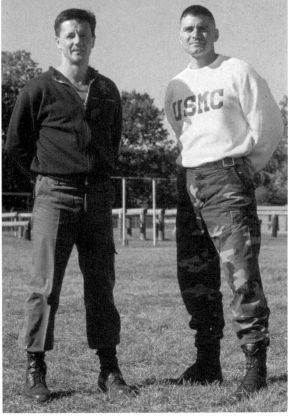

A British Royal Marine, Warrant Officer Second Class (WO2) Andrew Burns served as Physical Training Advisor (PTA) to the Commanding Officer (CO) at OCS from 1996 to 1998 as part of an ongoing instructor exchange program between the US and Great Britain.

WO2 Burns joined the Royal Marines in September 1978. On completion of basic training he was drafted to 42 Commando Royal Marines and served in K Company as a rifleman.

During his six years with 42 Commando he served in the Falkland Islands Campaign, took part in a four month tour to South Armagh in Northern Ireland and was deployed to Norway for six Arctic winters.

In 1984, he attended the junior command course and was promoted to Corporal in 1985. Once promoted he volunteered for specialist PT training and completed his 19-week PT 2 course in September 1985. During the course he qualified as a ski instructor, canoe coach and rock climbing leader. He then spent three years at the Commando Training Center training recruits.

In 1988, he was drafted to 45 Commando in Scotland. Here he served as a section commander and completed another tour of duty in Belfast, Northern Ireland. He also took part in two more Arctic deployments.

In 1990, he returned to the Commando Training Center for his Senior Command Course, and promotion to Sergeant soon followed. The next 12 months were spent training young officers.

From 1991 to 1993, he served with the Royal Navy at their PT School in Portsmouth, England. Here he was responsible for running a 25-week physical training course for young navy personnel who aspired to become physical training instructors.

From 1993 to 1994, he returned to the Commando Training Center and the Royal Marines Physical Training School. Here he ran all PT courses. His last draft before coming to OCS was at the Royal Marine School of Music, Deal, where he was the Colour Sergeant Unit PTI advisor.

He attended the Advance Command Course in January 1997 and on his return to the UK will move to 40 Commando Royal Marines to take up the post of Sergeant Major.

W02 Burns is married. He and his wife Gail have two daughters, Victoria and Laura.

Sergeant Baldemar Benavidez

In April 1995, Sgt. Baldemar Benavidez was assigned to the Marine Corps Combat Development Command, Quantico, Virginia, at Officer Candidate School. Here he was a Fire Team Leader and later a

Squad Leader for the Communications and Demonstration Platoon.

In January 1997 he was reassigned to the Physical Training Section as a Physical Training Instructor. Sgt. Benavidez has since trained five companies of Officer Candidates in physical fitness.

Sgt. Benavidez joined the Marines in 1991. Upon completion of recruit training, he served in Echo Battery, 10th Marines, 2nd Marine Division as a cannoneer, and performed all duties as required by an artillery gun section.

During his four years with Echo Battery, 10th Marines, he served on two six-month deployments, the first to Okinawa and the second with the 22nd Marine Expeditionary Unit in Bosnia and later Somalia. Additionally he participated in numerous live fire exercises to including a two-month

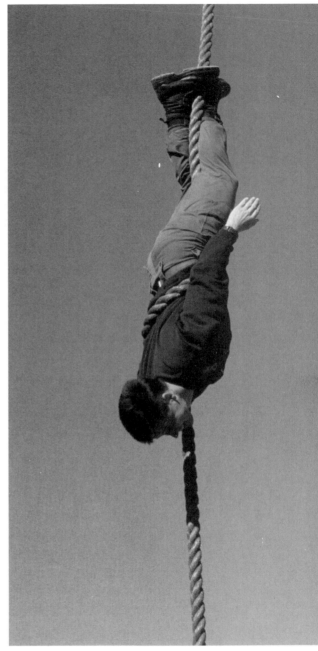

Andrew Burns demonstrates advanced rope descent technique. Don't try this at home!

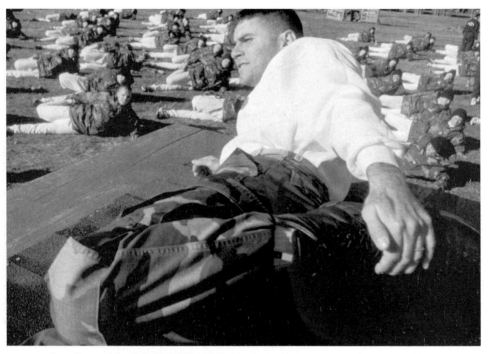

Sgt. Benavidez leads a PT session.

CAX (Combined Arms Exercise) in Twenty-Nine Palms, California and others in Fort Bragg, North Carolina.

Sergeant Benavidez has never received less than a first class rating on the Marine Corps PFT and has received 11 certificates of Physical Fitness Achievement.

Sergeant Benavidez is married. He and his wife Judith have two daughters, Catherine and Gabriella.

CLOSE-UP: THE STAMINA COURSE

Please Note: Obstacle courses are a staple of Marine Corps Physical Training. The challenge presented by the obstacles assists in developing and testing basic physical skills. In many combat situations, success will depend upon a Marine's ability to perform one or more of these skills, often while fully weighed down with gear and physically fatigued. The following obstacle courses are part of the physical readiness training of Marine Corps officers.

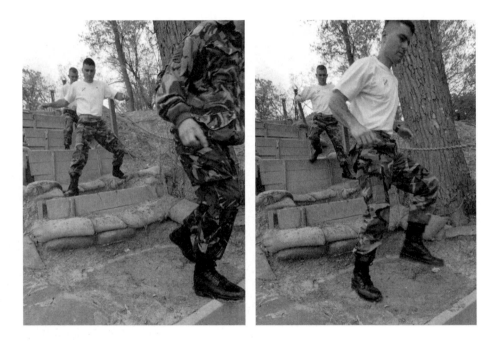

The first challenge is an **UPHILL SPRINT**. Using the steep, wide steps, jump down to the bottom of the hill. Now that you're there, turn and sprint back up the hill and jump the low hurdle.

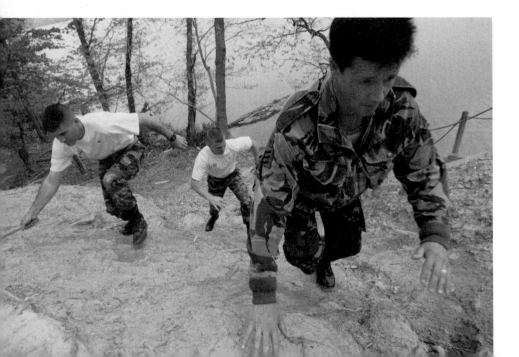

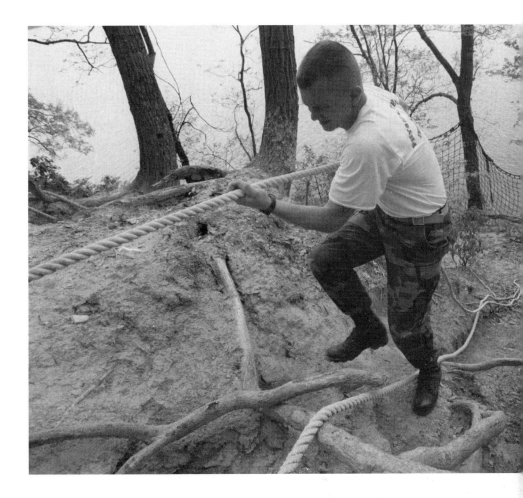

Next is the **CLIFF CLIMB**. At the bottom of the hill select a rope. Grasp the rope with both hands. Pull hand under hand, while using your legs for power.

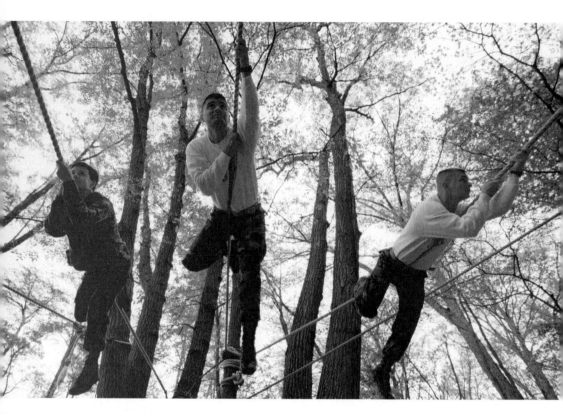

The **COMMANDO CRAWL** is accomplished by lying on top of the rope and hooking one leg over the rope with the other leg hanging down. Pull yourself forward, hand under hand, while pushing with the leg that is hooked over the rope. After reaching the end of the rope, release your hands and drop to the ground while bending your knees.

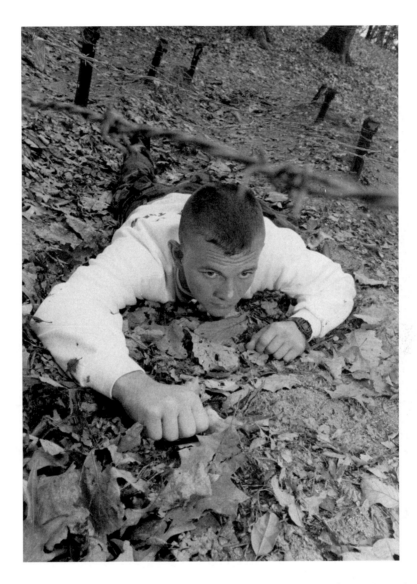

The **UPHILL LOW CRAWL** is negotiated by getting down in a low crawl position, keeping your head and buttocks down, while crawling under the barbed wire. Propel yourself forward by bending the knee of one leg and pushing with the inside edge of your boot. At the same time, move your opposite arm forward and pull to the rear. Keep your body low as you alternate this motion from side to side with your arms until the obstacle is cleared.

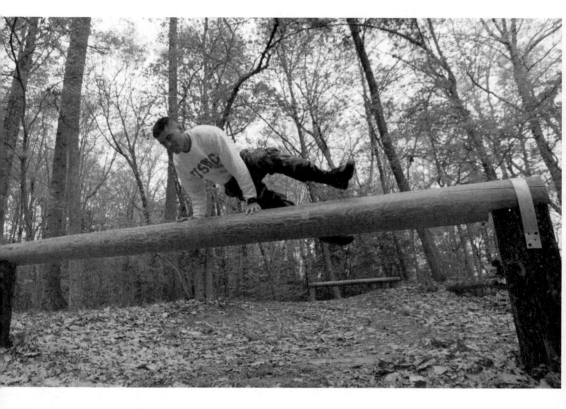

Next come a series of log obstacles. Go up and over each. **VAULTING** is the technique used to overcome these low barriers. Approach the logs at an angle. The hand on the side next to the obstacle is placed on top of the obstacle. With a straight arm, push your body weight upward. At the same time, throw your leg on the side next to the log over the top, followed by your other leg. Land with your weight on your leading leg first, then regain balance on both legs. Use your free arm all the while to help maintain your balance. And remember to keep moving!

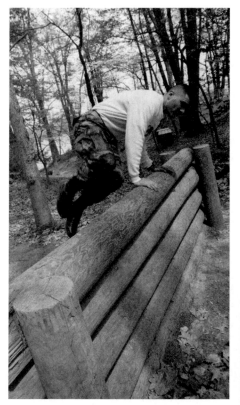

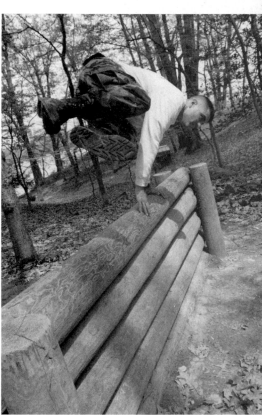

There are a number of vaulting obstacles, all in a row, including the medium vault, the wire, the high vault, the log vaulting wall, and the two high vaults. Pictured are the medium vault and the log vaulting wall.

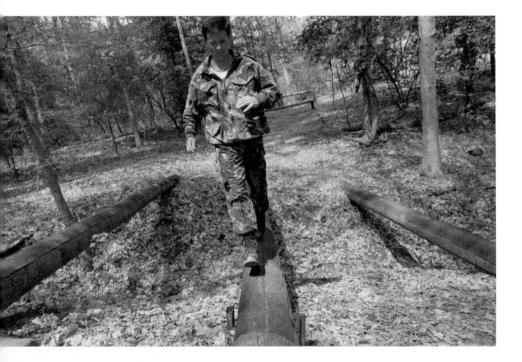

BALANCE LOGS are a real challenge. Balancing your body while walking and running on a narrow object is a skill that requires practice and confidence. Place your feet on the log, hold your arms to the sides about shoulder level, and fix your eyes on an object about 15 feet ahead. Try not to look at your feet as you walk down the log, placing one foot in front of the other in the center of the beam. Use your arms to help maintain balance.

The Balance Logs are followed by another **WIRE** obstacle. This time roll under the wire and log. This is followed by a **MEDIUM VAULT** and **HIGH VAULT**.

Roll under the log on the **LOW CRAWL HURDLE**.

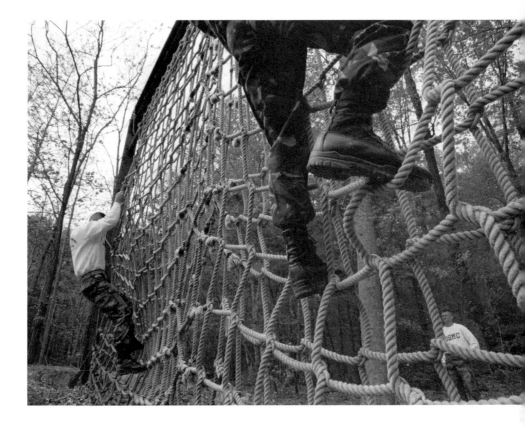

Finally you are at the **CARGO NET**. Reach the top by grabbing the vertical ropes with your hands and climbing on the horizontal ropes with your feet. Cross the top bar and climb down the other side. You're done!

CLOSE-UP: CONFIDENCE COURSE

T he men of the Combat Demonstration Platoon (CDP) were able to provide us with a fast paced run through the USMC OCS Confidence Course. The Confidence Course is an awesome challenge to anyone, yet to the men of the CDP it's all in a day's work. They train solely to demonstrate this course and others for members of the media, VIPs, and other distinguished visitors to Quantico.

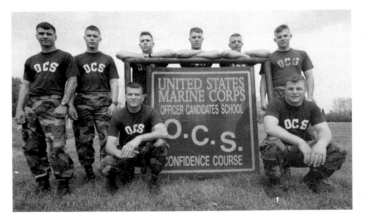

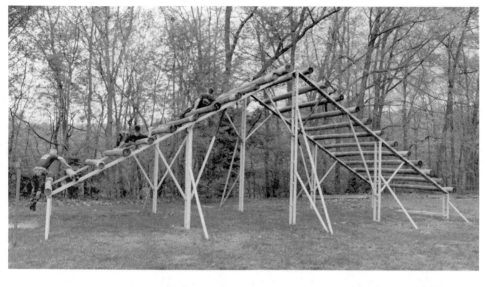

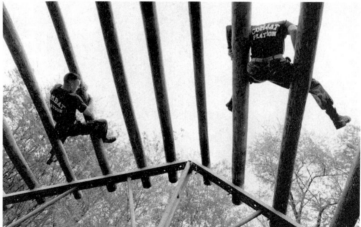

THE WEAVER

Mount the first log, go under the second, and over the third. Continue to weave through the obstacle, going over the logs that are painted yellow and under the unpainted logs. The top two logs on each side of the obstacle are painted yellow. Upon reaching the top yellow log, stand up and walk carefully to the opposite yellow log and begin your descent in the same manner.

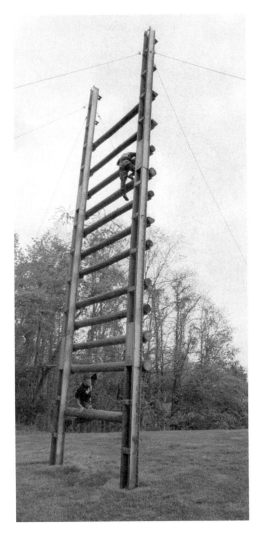

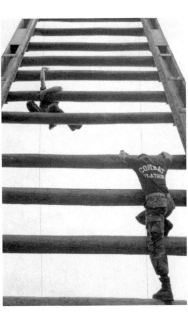

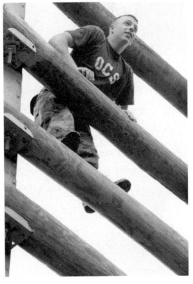

THE CONFIDENCE CLIMB

Climb up the right half of this over-sized ladder. Upon reaching the top, change sides by crossing over the yellow painted log. Lower yourself carefully by climbing down the left half of the ladder. Though it's tempting, don't use the steel uprights for support!

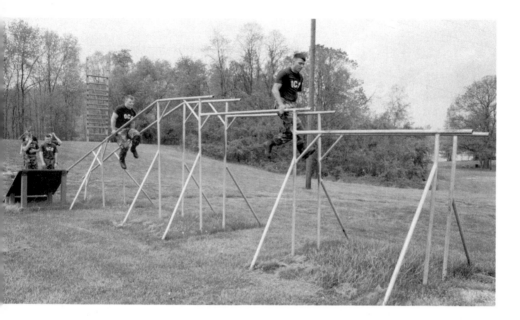

THE ARM WALK

This obstacle is accomplished like a moving dip. Here's how: Stand between the rails. Walk forward until the rails are even with your waist. Now grab the rails, jump up, and extend your arms, locking your elbows. Move forward and up the incline,

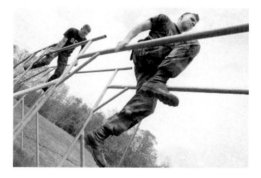

supporting your body on your extended arms. While moving forward on your right arm, flex your right knee. While moving forward on your left arm flex your left knee, and so on. The resulting movements will be similar to those of riding a bicycle. To move to the lower levels, shift your weight to one hand on the lower level. Keep moving to the end of the rails, perform one stationary dip to show everyone you're not the least bit tired, and vault off. Ooh Rah!

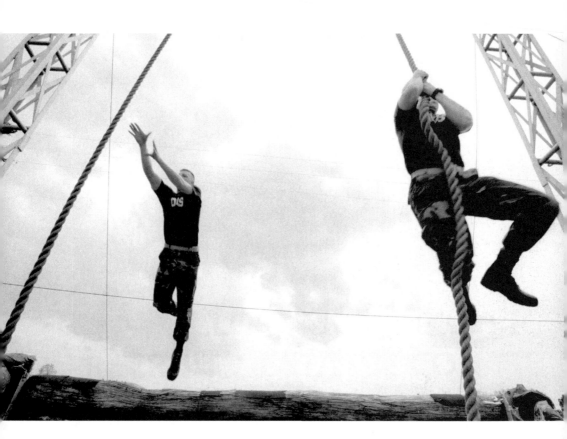

SWING AND JUMP

From a running start, dive out from the top of the incline and grasp the rope. While swinging forward your momentum will carry you to the far side. Fortunately, you are given two chances to successfully complete this obstacle.

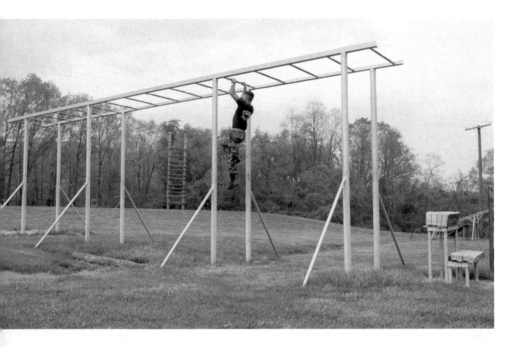

THE HORIZONTAL LADDER

Just like the old days in the playground? Far from it! Step up onto the top of the platform, jump up and grab the first rung. Negotiate all the remaining rungs hand-under-hand or hand-to-hand. Upon reaching the end drop off the obstacle.

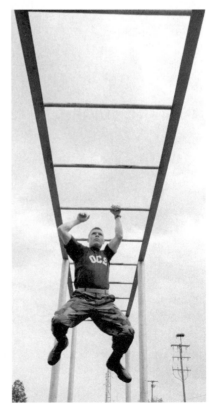

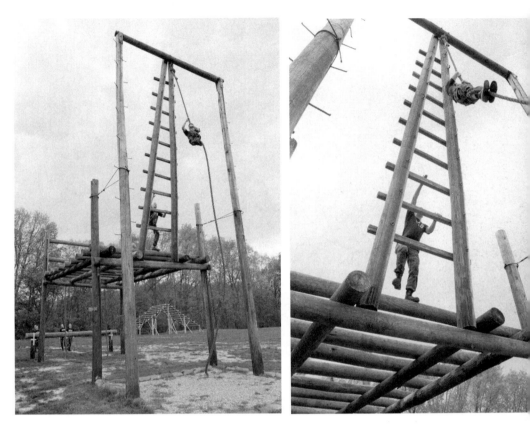

THE TOUGH ONE

When you look at it you think perhaps it should be called "The Impossible One." But it's not. You need to break it down into its components, tackle each in turn, and you've done it. This obstacle demands strength, balance, ingenuity, and plenty of confidence.

Step onto the low horizontal log. Climb the rope to reach the top. Pull yourself up to the platform. Walking slowly, traverse the platform by stepping on the individual logs lying across the supporting logs.

Upon reaching the rising ladder, climb up, making certain to keep one hand and one foot on the ladder at all times. When you've reached the second log from the top, sit down on that log and hold on with both arms around the uprights. Reach out with one foot and pull the rope toward you. Grasp the rope with one hand, ensuring

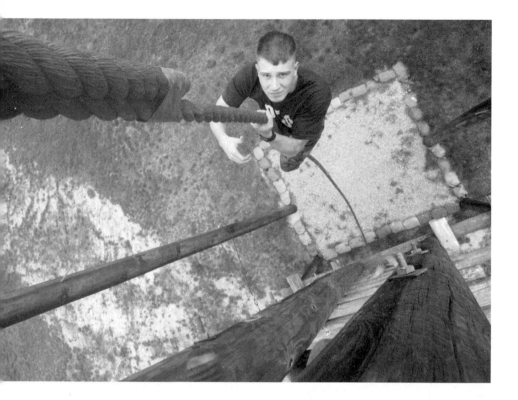

that the other hand is still on one of the upright supports. Wrap both feet around the rope and establish a good grip. Now with both hands and feet on the rope, swing out and lower yourself hand-over-hand in a controlled motion.

As you see, it's tough but not impossible!

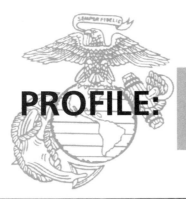

LIEUTENANT COMMANDER DENNIS J. ROCHEFORD, U.S.N. CHAPLAIN, THE BASIC SCHOOL

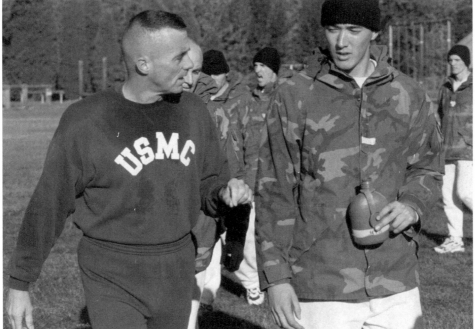

There are times when spiritual guidance, counseling, and encouragement are needed by the Officer Candidates. OCS demands a lot. Mentally, physically, spiritually. It's good to know that there is someone to talk to, someone who will listen.

Chaplain Rocheford grew up in Massachusetts and joined the Marine Corps in 1967. After graduation from recruit training at Parris Island, SC, Chaplain Rocheford joined "A" Company, 1st Battalion,

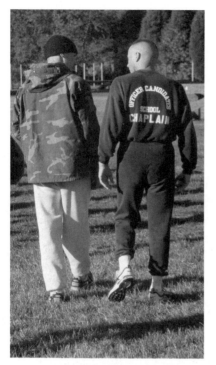

1st Marines as a rifleman and served from December 1967 until January 1969 in the Republic of Vietnam. Chaplain Rocheford participated in combat operations in Hue City, Khe San and DaNang. He was awarded a Navy Commendation Medal with Combat "V" for his service. His citation read in part that "Corporal Rocheford repeatedly distinguished himself by his courage and composure under fire. On 15 February…in the battle for Hue City, Corporal Rocheford's unit came under intense enemy rocket and automatic weapons fire. Realizing the seriousness of the situation he unhesitatingly exposed himself to the hostile fire as he skillfully directed mortar fire on the enemy position."

Upon return to the United States, Chaplain Rocheford served with 2nd Battalion, 2nd Marines at Camp Lejeune, NC and finally finished out his Marine Corps service as a Sergeant at Guantanamo Bay, Cuba. He then attended the University of Massachusetts, graduating in 1973 with a Bachelor of Arts degree. This schooling was soon followed by a Masters in Theology from St. John's Seminary in 1977 and another Masters in Religious Education from Boston College in 1984.

After 11 years of service as a parish priest in Worcester, M.A., Chaplain Rocheford entered the Chaplains Corps and began an 11-year stretch serving with the Marine Corps. During this period he's been assigned as the Chaplain for the Command Element of 22 Marine Expeditionary Unit (MEU), the battalion chaplain for 3rd Battalion, 8th Marines, the chaplain for the USS Wasp and finally at Quantico as the Chaplain for OCS, and then TBS.

Chaplain Rocheford is returning to the Worcester Diocese where he hopes to be the Commanding Officer of his own parish. We all wish him smooth seas and a following wind for every day of the future.

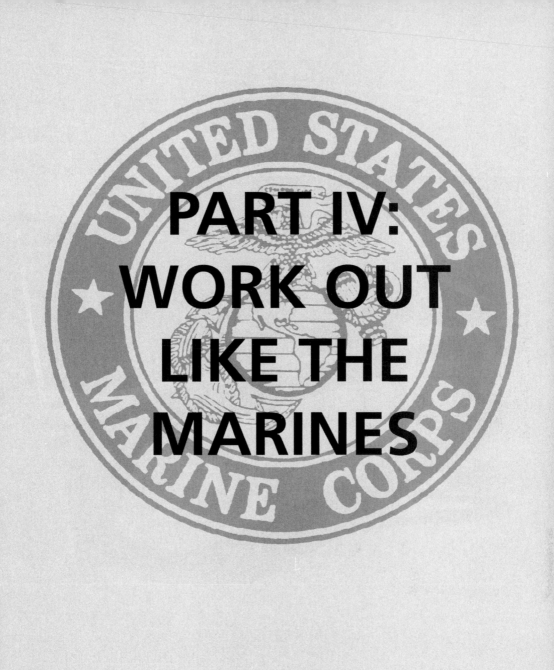

PART IV: WORK OUT LIKE THE MARINES

THE US MARINE CORPS DAILY 16 WORKOUT

INTRODUCTION

The Marine Corps has developed a uniquely effective fitness program consisting of a series of warmups, stretches, upper body, lower body, and abdominal exercises. This combination of exercises is designed to be performed anywhere a Marine goes: on a ship at sea, at the base, in the field. These exercises require no equipment and rely solely on one's own body weight for resistance. Together they are known as the "Daily 16".

The Daily 16 can be accomplished by men and women, Marines and civilians, young and old. The 16 exercises were selected by an expert committee consisting of sports medicine specialists, exercise physiologists, and kinesthesiologists. Kinesthiology is the study of human motion, blending the sciences of anatomy, physiology, biomechanics, and neurology.

THE DAILY 16

The Daily 16 consists of 8 stretches and 8 exercises preceded by a warm-up routine. The stretches and exercises are organized into "cards." These cards are actual laminated cards carried by the Drill Instructors (D.I.'s) who lead the exercise routines. There is one warm-up card, two stretching cards, and three exercise cards. Each day one stretch card and one exercise card are chosen. In Marine Corps training, the selection of the card is at the discretion of the Drill Instructor. If a Marine is on his or her own, the selection can be made by the individual. The Daily 16 is an effective total body workout if performed regularly.

The sequence begins with two minutes of warm-up exercises to get your body ready for the workout. You'll then move on to stretching.

Choose one of the two stretching cards and perform each stretch as described and illustrated in the following pages. Hold each stretch for 10 seconds. The goal of this stretch sequence is to warm up. When performing the stretches, don't bounce. Stretch in a static hold and try to relax the rest of your body as much as possible. You want the muscles that you're trying to stretch to be as relaxed as possible. Keep your breathing regular and relaxed—try not to hold your breath while stretching.

Continue by selecting one of the three exercise cards and performing five repetitions of each exercise. Why only five repetitions? Because this is still part of the overall warm-up. You will be exercising at higher repetitions soon enough!

You'll then move to the main physical fitness event. In Marine Corps training, the main fitness event might be a squad ability run, the obstacle course, or the circuit course. If at sea, you might run on the flight deck, or use one of the stationary bikes or treadmills. If on base, you could swim laps in the pool. If you are not going through a predetermined training program, your main fitness event could be a run, bike ride, or swim, for example. The main fitness event should last about 20 minutes.

Then it's back to the same exercise card you used to warm up— only now it's the real thing! Perform the sequence in sets of 10 to 20 reps, depending upon your fitness level. Choose a level that is challenging for you. Your Drill Instructor most certainly will have a plan for you if you are undergoing Marine Corps training. Suffice to say that will be challenging. You might repeat the sets and reps twice or three times to increase the intensity of your workout. Whatever you do, keep to the sequence to achieve your desired fitness goals.

When you're finished, it's time for a final stretch. This time you're stretching for flexibility and cool down. Return to the stretch card of the day and this time hold each stretch for 30 seconds. You're done!

DAILY 16
WORKOUT SUMMARY

Warm-up Card	Perform for 2 minutes
Stretch Card	Hold each stretch for 10 seconds
Exercise Card	5 repetitions each for warm-up
Main Fitness Event	20 minutes minimum: run, swim, bike
Exercise Card	10-20 repetitions minimum each exercise
Stretch Card	Hold each stretch for 30 seconds

THE DAILY 16 WORKOUT CARDS

WARM-UP CARD
START Double Time in Place
Punch to the Front
Punch to the Sky
Arm Circles
END Double time in Place
Neck ROTATIONS
Trunk Rotations
Knee and Ankle Rotations

STRETCHING CARD 1
triceps stretch
upper back stretch
chest stretch
iliotibial band (itb) stretch
calf stretch
hip and back stretch
modified hurdler stretch
groin stretch

STRETCHING CARD 2
triceps stretch
posterior shoulder stretch
shoulder and neck stretch
calf stretch
hip and back stretch
iliotibial band (itb)
        stretch (Lying)
quadriceps stretch
hamstrings stretch

EXERCISE CARD 1
pushups
dirty dogs
crunches
wide pushups
back extensions
elbow to knee crunches
lunges
side straddle hops

EXERCISE CARD 2
pushups
dirty dogs
crunches
dive bombers
donkey kicks
side crunches
lunges
steam engines

EXERCISE CARD 3
eight count body
        builder pushups
side leg raises
elbow to knee crunches
dive bombers
hip adduction
side crunches
prone flutter kicks
steam engines

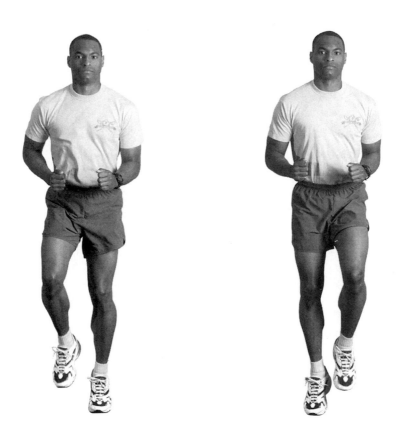

DOUBLE TIME IN PLACE

Start off with smaller steps, and as you continue running begin to bring your knees up higher. Relax, and let your muscles get loose and warm before moving on to the next warm-up activity. Double time in place for 15 seconds, then...

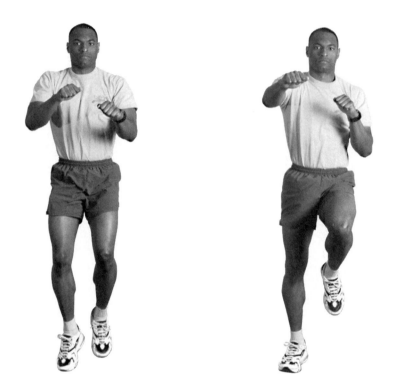

...PUNCH TO THE FRONT

While increasing the intensity of your double time in place, add in punches to the front for 15 seconds. This helps to warm up your upper body.

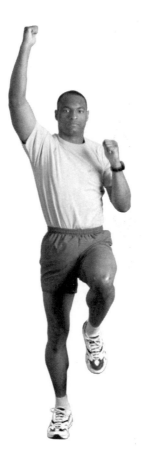

PUNCH TO THE SKY

This is another way to get your upper body warmed up and ready for exercising. While maintaining the double time, punch skyward for 15 seconds.

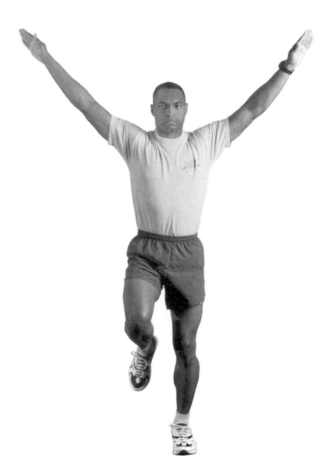

ARM CIRCLES

While running in place, start rotating your arms in large circles, first forward and then backward. Be sure to keep your arms straight! Your arms should form a "V" as shown. Perform arm circles for 15 seconds.

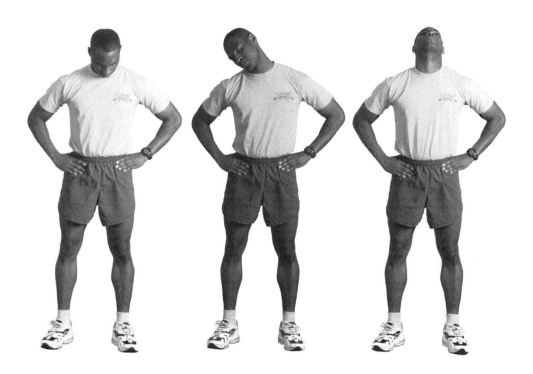

NECK ROTATIONS

Stop the double time in place for this exercise. Rotate your neck to the right, then to the left. Be very gentle! Your neck and spine are highly prone to injury and you should make certain that any stretches and exercises which use the neck and spine are done at an easy pace.

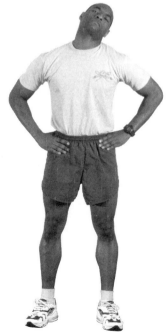

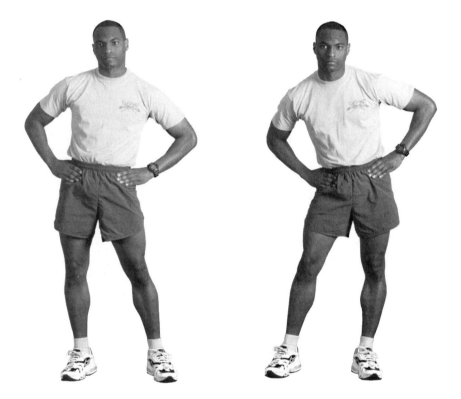

TRUNK ROTATIONS

This exercise is designed to warm up your body' s midsection, or trunk. Start by swinging your hips in a circular motion. This permits more mobility in the trunk and loosens up your abdominal and lower back area. Again, be gentle with these motions. You are NOT keeping a hula-hoop on your hips! Gentle, gentle, gentle.

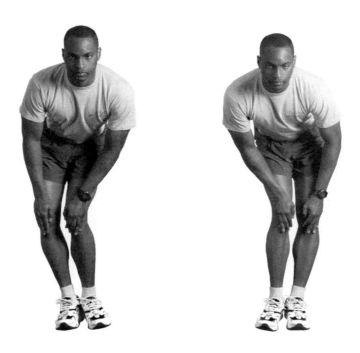

KNEE AND ANKLE ROTATIONS

Place your hands on your knees, place your feet together, and rotate your knees and ankles. Rotate clockwise, then counter clockwise.

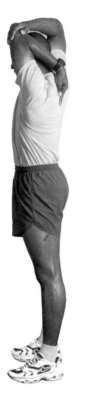
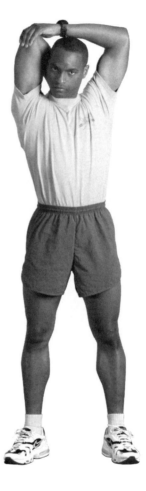

TRICEP STRETCH

Pull your left arm behind your head and reach down towards your shoulder blades with your left hand as shown. You can pull on your left elbow with your right hand for added stretch. Repeat for the right triceps.

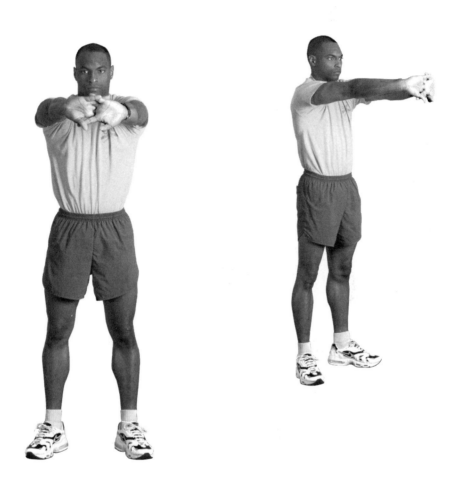

UPPER BACK STRETCH

Lace your fingers together in front while reaching forward. Try to stretch your shoulder blades while rolling your shoulders as far forward as possible. This stretches the muscles in the upper part of your back between your shoulder blades.

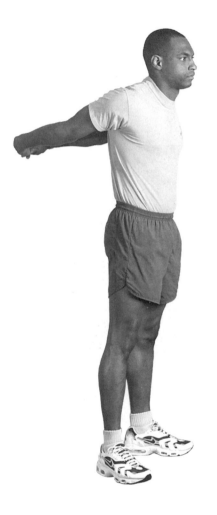

CHEST STRETCH

Clasp your hands behind your back and lift your arms straight back. This stretches muscles on the front part of the chest and a portion of your shoulders. This is also known as "the swimmer stretch."

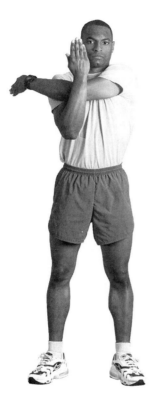

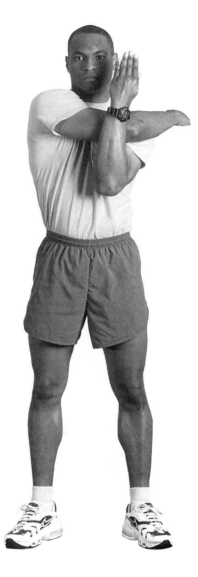

POSTERIOR SHOULDER STRETCH

Extend your left elbow across your body and place your right hand as shown. Keep your shoulders level for maximum benefit and to avoid injury. Switch arms and repeat.

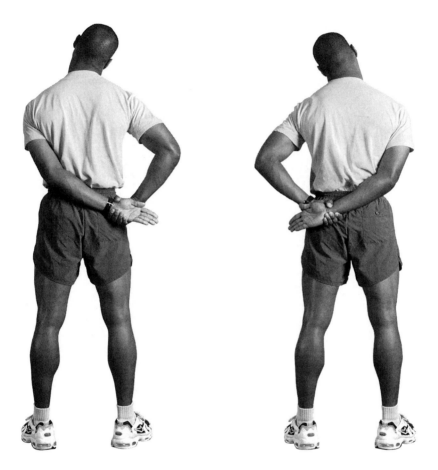

SHOULDER AND NECK STRETCH

Tilt your head to the right while pulling your left arm across your back as shown. You should feel this stretch on the top of your shoulder and into your neck as you work the trapezius and middle deltoid muscles. Repeat with your right arm across your back and your neck tilted to the left.

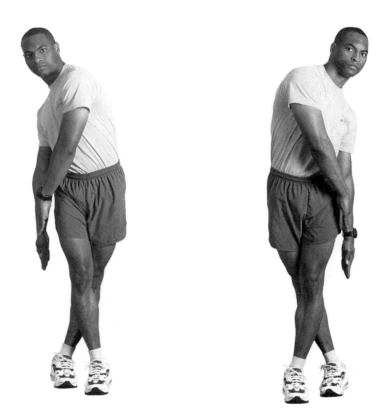

STANDING ILIOTIBIAL BAND (ITB) STRETCH

The ITB is essentially a tendon—a band of connective tissue—which runs the length of your thigh, crossing over the knee on the side. The ITB is most often injured from running. This ITB stretch will help prevent that kind of injury. The Standing ITB Stretch, in particular, isolates the ITB better than other ITB stretches.

Cross your left leg behind your right and bend down to the right, throwing your hips out to the left. You' ll feel this stretch in your left hip. Switch sides and repeat with the opposite leg.

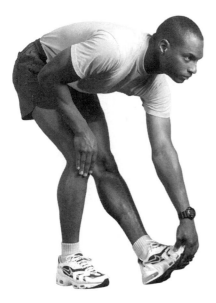

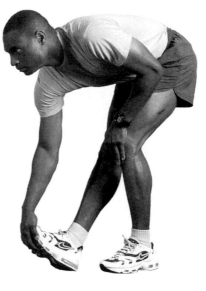

CALF STRETCH

Bend your right leg as shown and place your weight on it. Extend your left leg in front, keeping your left knee straight. While bending down, pull up on your left toes with your hand. Your left foot should be flexed. Feel the stretch in your left calf. Repeat with the right leg.

This stretch can be done with walls or steps to lean against, but out in the field there generally aren't walls for Marines to lean on, nor are there steps to put your foot on.

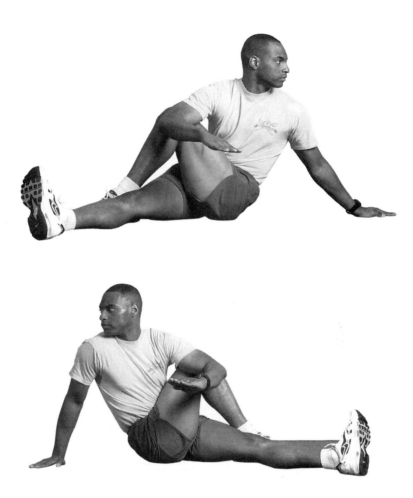

HIP AND BACK STRETCH

This is another iliotibial band (ITB) stretch. Sitting down, cross your left leg over your right, and push your left knee to the right with your right elbow, at the same time rotating your lower back as far as possible to the left. Keep your right leg straight out in front of you. Repeat with the right leg.

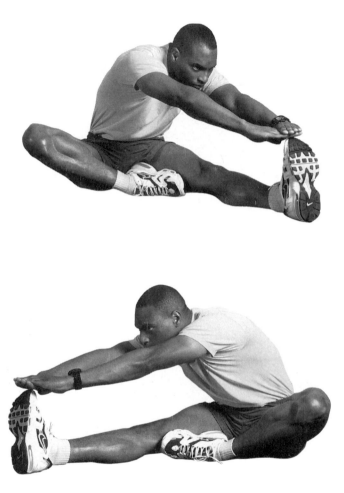

MODIFIED HURDLER STRETCH

Take your right leg and tuck it into the inside of your left thigh.
Reach down toward your left foot as far as possible. It' s very important to keep your left knee straight as you do this. You' ll feel this
primarily in your hamstring muscles, located in the back of your upper thigh, as well as through the medial muscles and up into your
back. Repeat on the other leg.

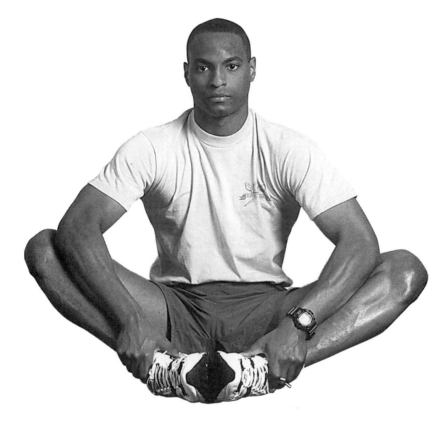

GROIN STRETCH

This is also known as the butterfly stretch. Tuck your heels in towards your groin. Try to bring your knees to the ground by pushing
down on them gently with your elbows.

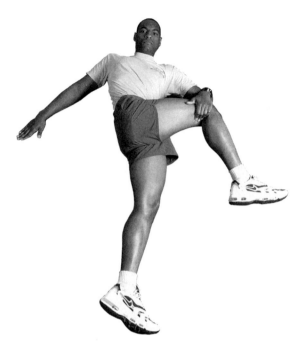

LYING DOWN ILIOTIBIAL BAND (ITB) STRETCH

Lie on your back. Using your left hand, pull your right leg over your body with your knee bent at a 90-degree angle, as demonstrated above. Your right hand should be straight and placed opposite the direction of your stretch. Repeat with the other leg.

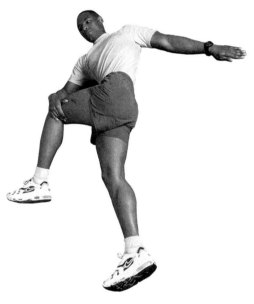

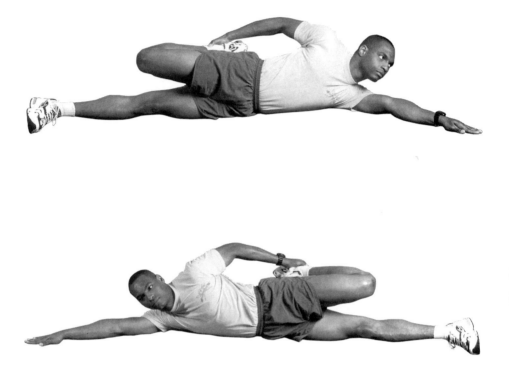

QUADRICEP STRETCH

Lying on your right side, pull your left heel into your buttocks and your left knee backward. Repeat with the right leg. This stretch may also be done while standing. The quadriceps are the muscles of your thigh. The primary function of the quadriceps is to extend the knee.

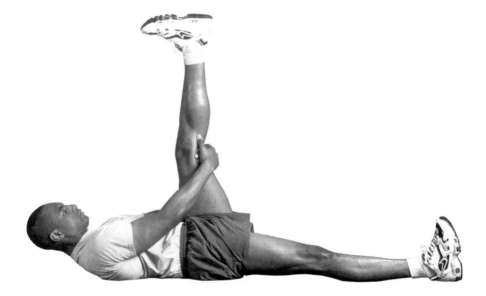

HAMSTRING STRETCH

The hamstrings are the muscles located in the back of your thigh. Lie on your back and raise your left leg as far up as possible using the muscles in your hip. Stretch your hamstrings further by placing your hands behind the knee and applying gentle pressure. Try to keep your knee as straight as possible. Repeat with the opposite leg.

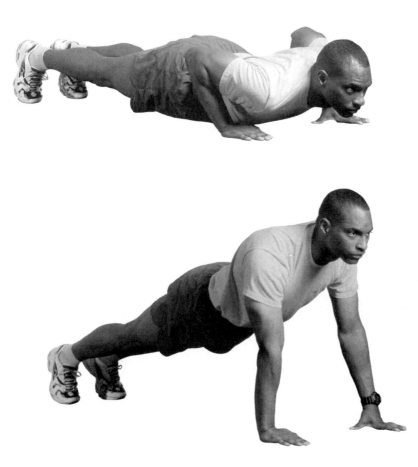

PUSHUPS

Marines love doing pushups. Hundreds of them. If you're training to be a Marine, and are expected to crank out 50 pushups in two minutes, be prepared to do 75. Learn to love the classic pushup. Place your hands on the ground straight below your shoulders, keeping your back straight. Lower yourself slowly to a count of four. Return to the starting position and repeat. And repeat.

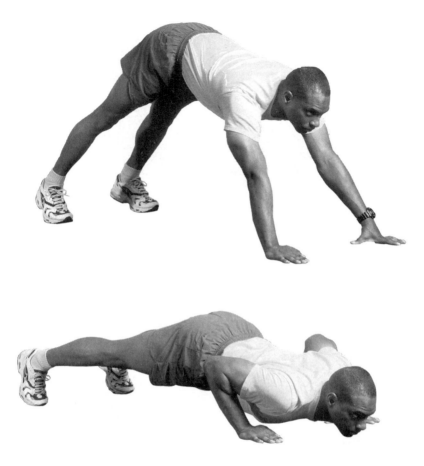

DIVE BOMBERS

Ever see the John Wayne film *The Flying Leathernecks*? Rent it some time, and while you are watching, you can crank out some Dive Bomber pushups. Start with your buttocks in the air and your shoulders back behind your hands. Your feet and hands should be spread a little more than shoulder width apart, but not as much as the wide pushups. With a smooth and controlled motion, lower yourself to the ground as shown and sweep your shoulders forward in front your hands. Reverse the motion to arrive at the beginning position.

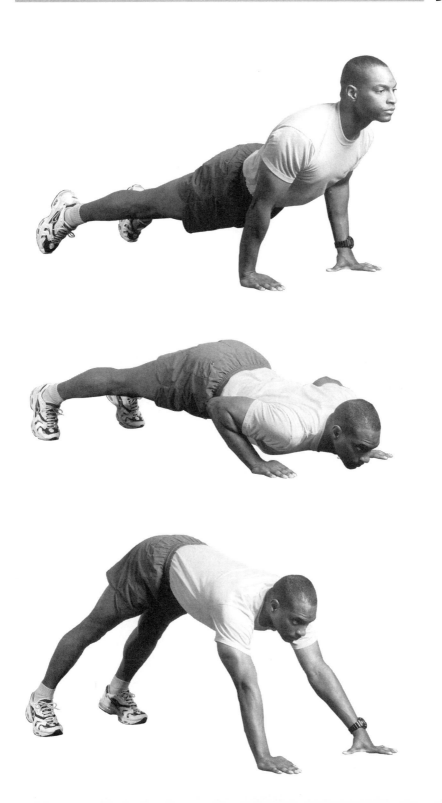

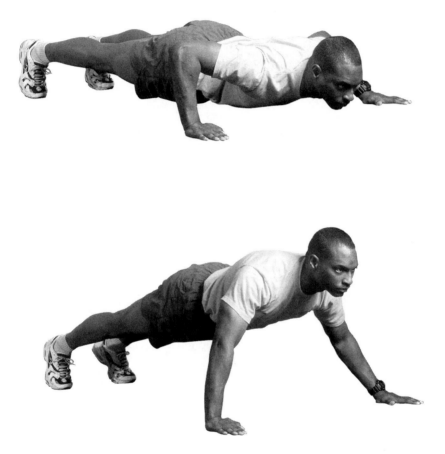

WIDE PUSHUPS

This is a variation of the classic pushup. This time, place your hands wider than shoulder width. Keeping your back straight, lower your-self in a controlled fashion to a count of four and return to the start-ing position. Repeat. The wide pushup works your chest muscles with greater intensity.

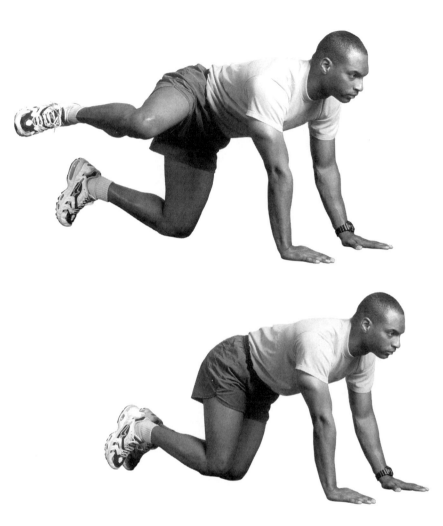

DIRTY DOGS

Dirty dogs, more commonly referred to as side leg lifts, work the hip abductors. Start by squatting on your hands and knees. Lift your right leg away from your body, bringing it to the height of your shoulder. Keep your leg straight out to the side, while maintaining a 90-degree angle with your knee. Bring your leg back down. Perform the specified number of repetitions on the right side, then repeat with the opposite leg.

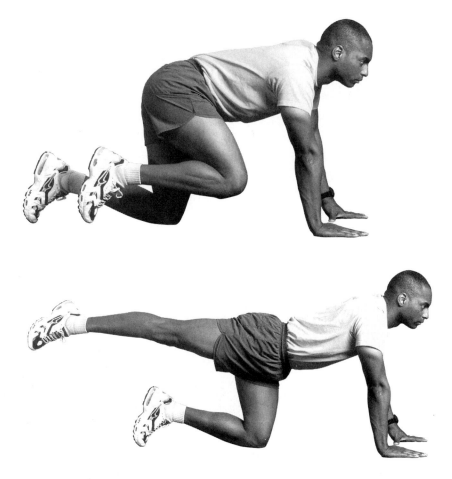

DONKEY KICKS

Squatting on your hands and knees, bring your right knee up towards your chest. Then push your leg behind you as shown, keeping your leg straight. Repeat for the specified number of repetitions, and then switch sides. This exercise works the hip extensors.

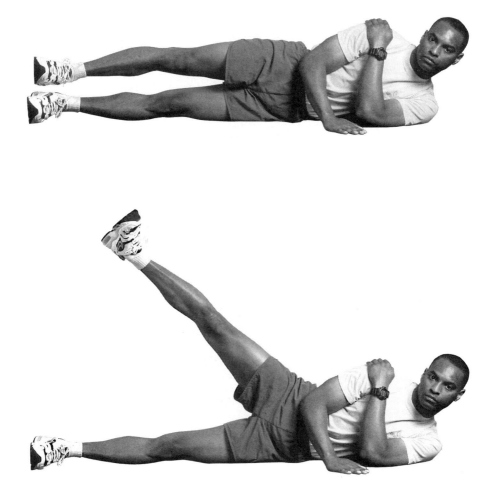

SIDE LEG RAISES

Lie on your right side with your body perpendicular to the ground. Bring your left leg straight up. Then bring it down again in a smooth motion. Keep your left knee and foot pointing straight forward as shown in the photograph. Repeat for the specified number of repetitions and switch sides.

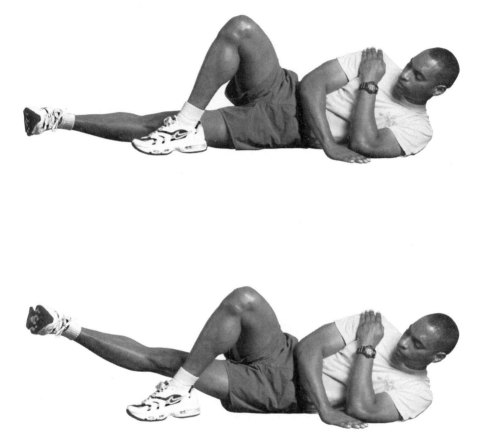

HIP ADDUCTION

This exercise benefits the muscles on the inside of your thigh. Lying on your left side with your right leg crossed over your left, raise your left leg upward while you squeeze your thighs together. Keep your knee and toes pointing forward. Your right foot should be flat on the floor. Repeat specified number of times on both sides.

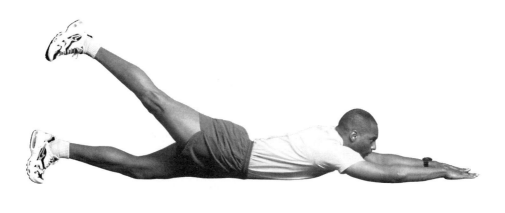

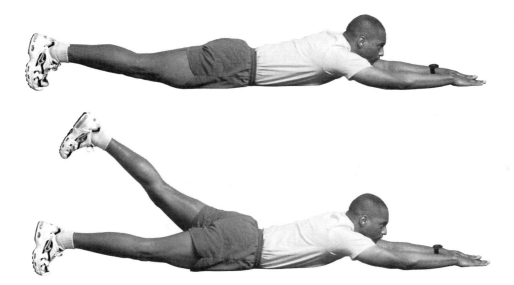

PRONE FLUTTER KICKS

Flutter kicks are another excellent hip extension exercise. Start off on your stomach with your arms in front of you. Raise one leg at a time. This works the muscles in your buttocks as well as your hamstrings—the muscle down the back of your thighs.

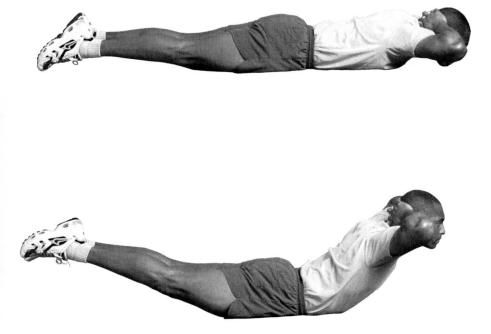

BACK EXTENSIONS

Lying on your stomach as shown, clasp your hands behind your head. Gently raise your upper body and legs off the ground and then lower yourself to the starting position. As with all exercises that incorporate the lower back, be careful not to exert too much stress while performing the required repetitions.

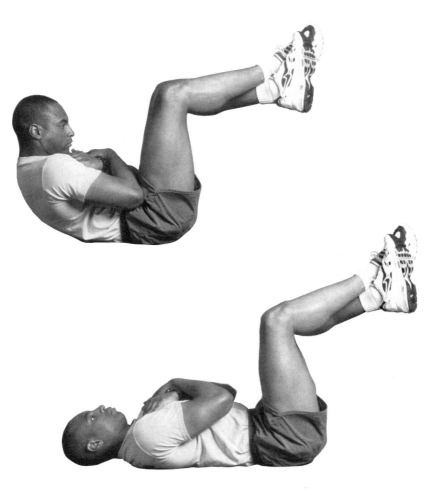

CRUNCHES

It's ab time! Lie on your back with your knees and hips at a 90-degree angle. Keep your feet elevated for this exercise. Cross your arms on your chest rather than placing your hands behind your head. This prevents you from pulling on your neck as you move upward. Lift your shoulders off the ground while your contract your stomach muscles, until your elbows touch your thighs. Return to the starting position and repeat.

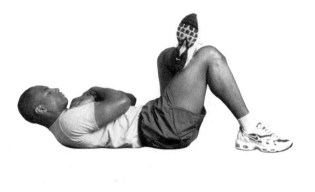

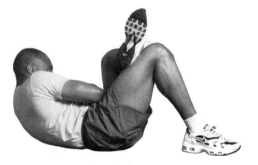

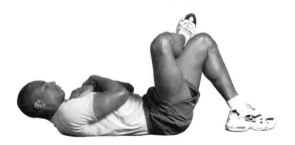

ELBOW-TO-KNEE CRUNCHES

Lying on the ground, place your left ankle on your right knee. Keep your hands folded across your chest as with the regular crunch. Lift your shoulders up as you rotate to bring your right elbow to your left thigh. This is an excellent exercise for strengthening and toning your side abdominal muscles, the obliques.

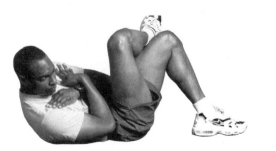

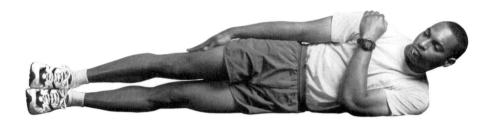

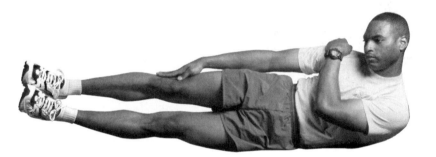

SIDE CRUNCHES

Start by lying on your left side. With your left arm crossed over your chest, grab your right shoulder. Keep your right arm straight along side your body as shown. Now, at the same time, lift your legs up off the ground and move your left shoulder upward as you slide your right hand along your torso toward your knee. Perform on both sides for the specified number of repetitions.

143

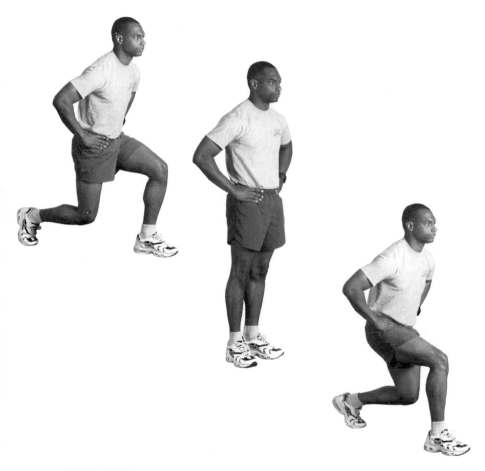

LUNGES

Start with your hands on your hips. To perform a proper lunge you should always keep your back straight and protected. With your left foot forward and your right behind, lower yourself by bending your right leg at the knee. Keep your front knee above your ankle as you drop down, and don't bend your left leg more than 90 degrees to avoid overstressing the knee joint. Use your left leg's thigh muscle to control the motion up and down. You will really feel this in your quadriceps. Repeat on both sides.

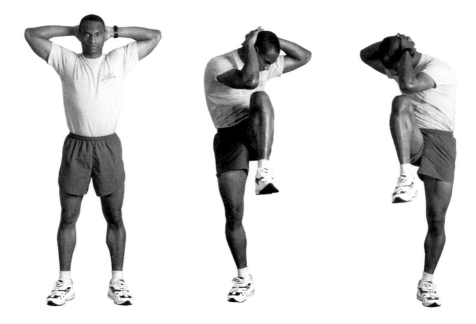

STEAM ENGINES

Steam Engines, like the Side Straddle Hops, are a total body exercise. Start with your hands behind your head, feet about shoulder width apart. Lower one elbow toward your opposite knee while bringing that knee up, so you are meeting in the middle as shown. This exercise is performed as a rapid continuous movement. It should take you approximately one second per side back and forth. Perform an equal number of repetitions on both sides.

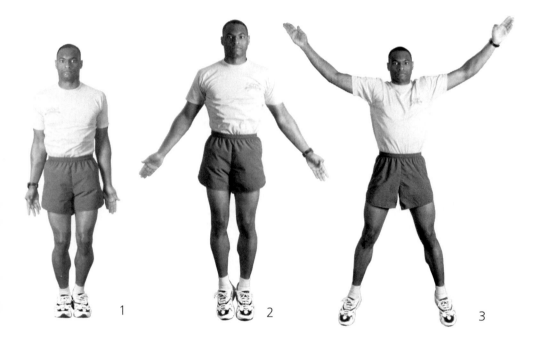

SIDE STRADDLE HOPS

Commonly known as Jumping Jacks, Side Straddle Hops are performed as follows: Begin with feet together and arms at your sides. As you jump up your feet should come apart and your hands should go over your head. As you land, bring your feet together and your hands together over your head. Side Straddle Hops are a great total body, cardio exercise.

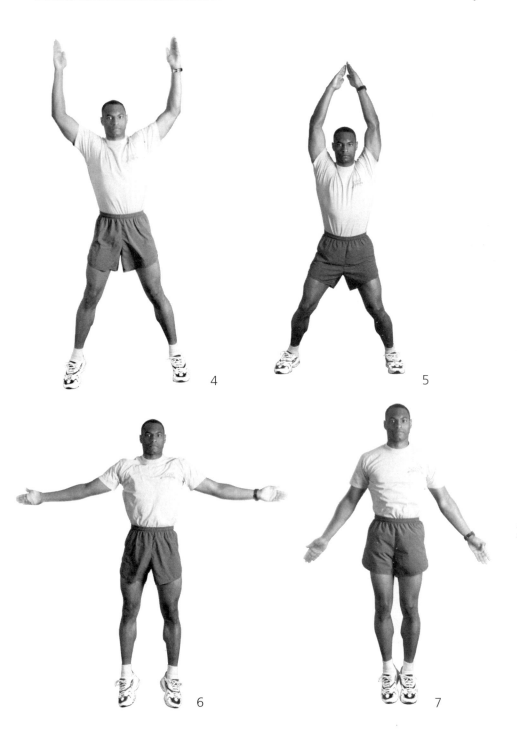

4

5

6

7

147

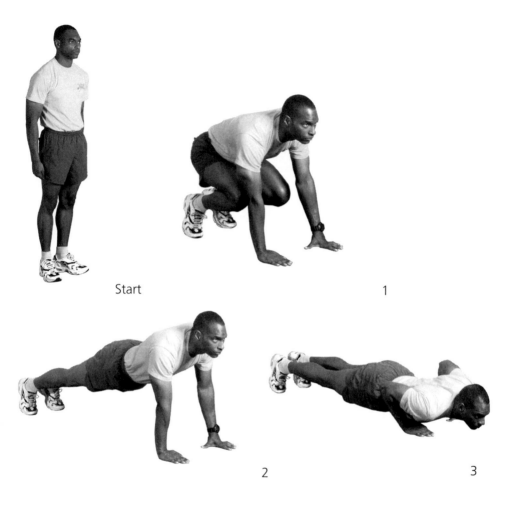

Start

1

2

3

EIGHT COUNT BODYBUILDERS

Stand at attention. On the first count, assume a squatting position with your hands on the ground and your knees bent. On the second count, kick your legs back. You will be in the "up" position of a pushup. On the third count lower yourself to the "down" position of a pushup. On four go "up". Five "down". Six "up". Seven, bring your knees in to the squat position again. On the count of eight, return to the "at attention" position. Repeat as required.

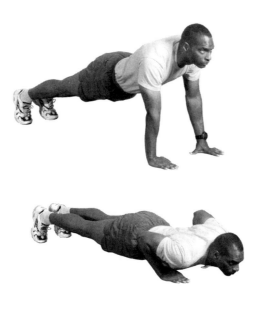

4

5

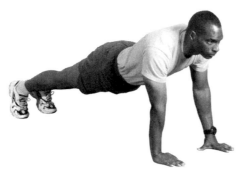

6

7

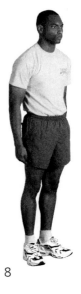

8

149

PROFILE:

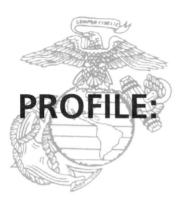

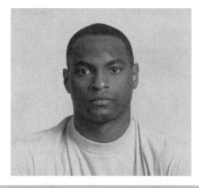

CHARLES L. ROLLINS
Staff Sergeant, United
States Marine Corps

Staff Sergeant Rollins was born and raised in Atlanta, Georgia where he graduated from Druid Hills High school and enlisted in the United States Marine Corps in 1986. His first assignment was at Camp Pendleton, California as a cook after completing Basic Cook School in Camp Johnson, North Carolina. In 1988, he was selected as Cook of the Quarter and in 1989 he was then asigned to Okinawa, Japan where he was promoted to Chief Cook at the messhall at Camp Kinser.

In 1990, Staff Sergeant Rollins participated in Operation Desert Shield/Desert Storm and in 1991 returned back to the states to Camp Lejeune, North Carolina where he soon deployed to Guantanimo Bay, Cuba for the Haitian migrants and was awarded a Citation for exceptional performance of duty while serving as a Food Service Specialist. From 1992 to 1994, Rollins was stationed with several units on the East Coast including Camp Geiger, North Carolina and Marine Corps Security Force Battalion in Norfolk, Virginia where he received yet another award for outstanding professionalism, going above and beyond the call of duty, by the International Food Service Executive Association Award (IFSEA - "Celebrate People").

In 1996, Rollins received orders to become a Drill Instructor and attended "D.I." school at Marine Corps Recruit Depot Parris Island. He then was assigned to the 3rd Recruit Training Battalion in Norfolk, Virginia and later became the Senior Drill Instructor for the Medical Rehabilitation Platoon where he currently is assigned.

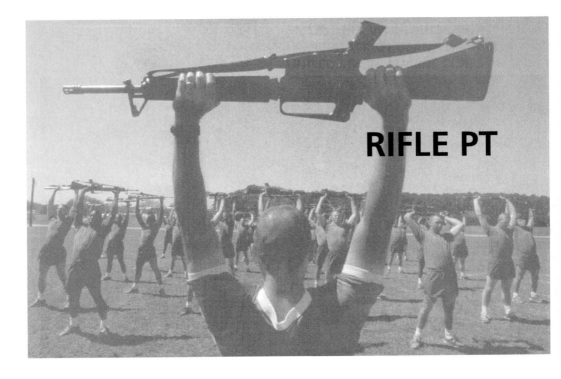

RIFLE PT

Rifle PT utilizes a tool that's very dear to the Marine—their weapon—as a source of resistance. In Marine Corps training, recruits use an M-16 rifle, which has a weight of 8.6 pounds, for these exercises. If you don't have access to a rifle, you can use just about anything that has a comparable weight, such as a ten-pound padded bar, soup cans, socks filled with sand, or hand weights.

Rifle exercises are conditioning exercises performed incorporating theweight of the rifle. The drill takes 15 minutes to complete. The objective of rifle drills is to exercise the arms, shoulders, and back muscles in order to develop strength and endurance, particularly in the upper body.

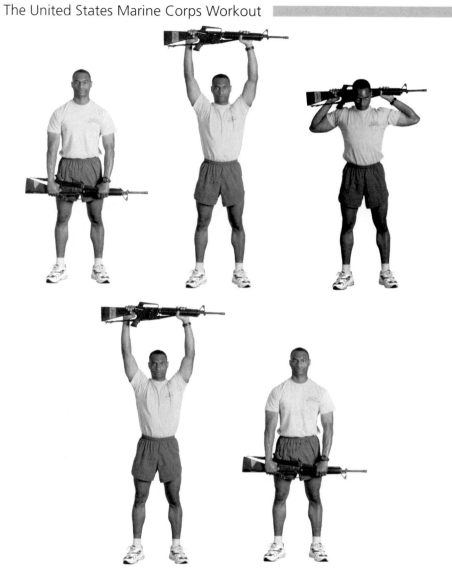

EXERCISE 1: FOREUP, BEHIND BACK

Start with your rifle downward and your feet together. This exercise is performed at a slow pace.

At the count of ONE: Swing your arms forward and upward to the overhead position. Inhale.

TWO: Lower your rifle to the back of your shoulders. Exhale.

THREE: Recover to position ONE and inhale.

FOUR: Recover to the starting position and exhale.

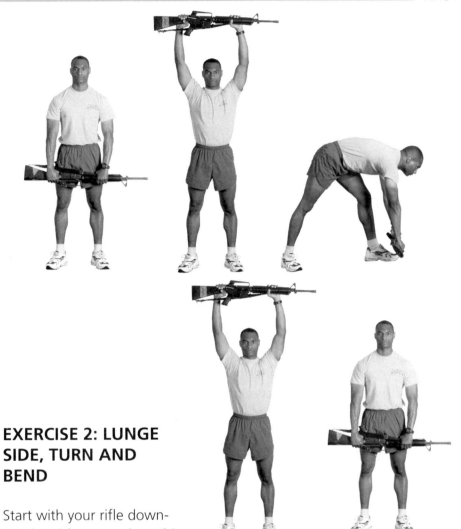

EXERCISE 2: LUNGE SIDE, TURN AND BEND

Start with your rifle downward and feet together. This time the exercise is done at a moderate pace. The Lunge Side Turn and Bend is an eight-count exercise. At the count of...

ONE: Lunge sidewards to your left, swing your rifle forward and upward to the overhead position.

TWO: Turn your torso to the left and bend forward over your left hip. At the same time, swing your rifle to a low horizontal position in front of your left ankle.

THREE: Recover to position ONE.

FOUR: Recover to the starting position.

FIVE, SIX, SEVEN, and EIGHT: Repeat the exercise on your right side.

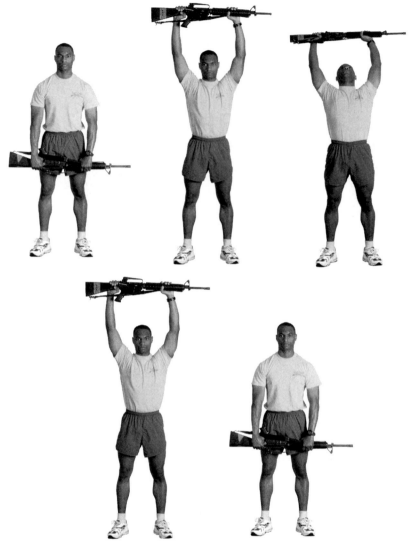

EXERCISE 3: FOREUP, BACK BEND

Starting with your rifle downward and your feet together. The pace is moderate.

At the count of...

ONE: Swing your arms forward and upward to the overhead position.

TWO: Gently bend backward as shown, emphasizing the bend in the upper back. Keep your head up and your knees straight.

THREE: Recover to position ONE.

154 FOUR: Recover to the starting position.

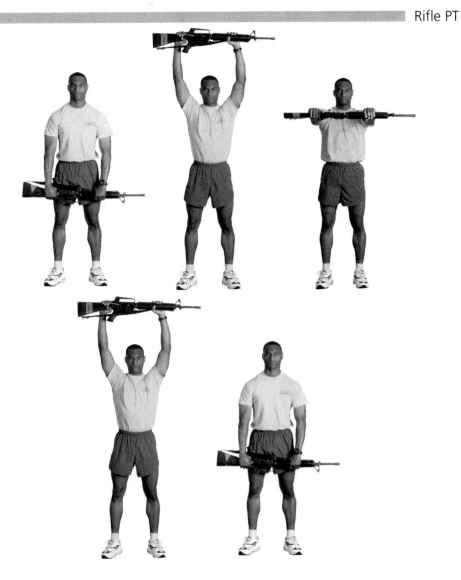

EXERCISE 4: UP AND FORWARD

Start with your rifle downward and your feet together. This time, the pace is fast.
At the count of...
ONE: Swing your arms forward and upward to the overhead position.
TWO: Swing your arms forward to shoulder level.
THREE: Recover to position ONE.
FOUR: Recover to the starting position.

155

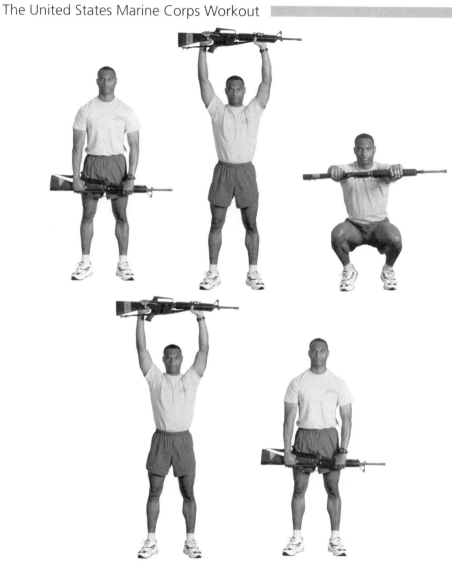

EXERCISE 5: FOREUP, FULL SQUAT

Start with your rifle downward and your feet about shoulder width apart. The pace for this exercise is moderate.

At the count of...

ONE: Swing your arms forward and upward to the overhead position.

TWO: Swing your arms down to shoulder level and assume a squatting position.

THREE: Recover to position ONE.

FOUR: Recover to the starting position.

WORKOUT SCHEDULES

There are an unlimited number of ways to combine the exercises found in this book. The key reminder: when it comes to fitness, there's no excuse not to do something!

We've assembled a few authentic Marine Corps workout routines to help organize your fitness program. They say "variety is the spice of life," and with your workouts the same holds true.

GET FIT GUIDELINES

WARMUP Always warmup before any strenuous workout to increase both the flexibility of your muscles and your heart rate. This prepares your body for the increased stress of physical exercise. When you properly prepare your muscles, tendons, ligaments and heart for a workout, exercise is more efficient and the potential for injury is reduced. To warmup you should walk or jog in place or perform calisthenic exercises like jumping jacks for two to three minutes.

When you're done, it's time to stretch.

STRETCH Stretch to the point of tightness and hold that position for 15 seconds. Do not bounce when stretching. Bouncing initiates the stretch reflex, causing muscles to tighten rather than relax. It also increases the chance of injury to muscles and joints.

COOL-DOWN You can recover faster from any sustained physical activity by continuing to participate in some type of low-intensity exercise such as walking after you are finished exercising. This helps prevent pooling of blood in the legs. As well, the contractions of the legs during walking will help return blood to your heart. Cool-down exercises also help to prevent muscle soreness that may follow infrequent physical activity.

UPPER BODY DEVELOPMENT (UBD) PYRAMIDS

The UBD pyramid consists of a series of sets of exercises, each containing pull-ups, pushups, chin-ups (or reverse grip pull-ups), and crunches. The combination is extremely effective for developing upper body strength and endurance. A pyramid starts with few repetitions, then increases with each set until the halfway point (the top of the pyramid). On the way down, repetitions decrease to the starting level. The pyramid is truly effective because it features a gradual warmup, peak effort, and a cool-down.

While performing a set, make certain you go from one exercise to the next without resting in between. Between sets take a minute break. The number of sets performed depends upon your fitness level. You should perform enough sets to produce an overload, or muscle fatigue.

The idea is to use the muscle to maximum capacity, thereby increasing muscle strength. When you've reached your limits you've used your current muscle capacity. This does not have to hurt. Your muscles will let you know when they can't operate any further.

In order to progress and increase muscle strength, you must know your maximum capacity. Increasing repetitions of an exercise will help build strength and endurance. After doing pushups, for example, if you can only do a set of 10 pushups before you can't do any more, then you know that's your limit. Perform sets often and increase repetitions and you'll notice that after a few weeks, you may be able to do a set of 25 pushups before you reach muscle fatigue.

When you can't do any more repetitions, use negatives to complete the pyramid. A negative, or eccentric contraction, means that you use your body weight—and gravity—to gain benefit from the exercise. For example, a negative pushup starts in the "up" position. Slowly lower yourself to the "down" position in a controlled manner. You can perform negative pushups, pull-ups, crunches. The idea is to do what you can do!

Here's a sample pyramid workout:

	Pull-ups	*Pushups*	*Chin-ups*	*Crunches*
Set One	1	5	1	5
Set Two	2	10	2	10
Set Three	3	15	3	15
Set Four	2	10	2	10
Set Five	1	5	1	5
Totals	9	45	9	45

Another example of a UBD pyramid workout consists of pull-ups, pushups, and crunches. Start out with 1 pull-up and twice the number of pushups. Do your crunches in sets of 25 or 50 as shown. The crunches should be evenly distributed throughout the sets to allow your upper body to recover from time-to-time.

	Pull-ups	Pushups	Crunches
Set One	1	2	0
Set Two	2	4	0
Set Three	3	6	25
Set Four	4	8	0
Set Five	5	10	25
Set Six	6	12	0
Set Seven	7	14	50
Set Eight	7	14	0
Set Nine	6	12	0
Set Ten	5	10	25
Set Eleven	4	8	0
Set Twelve	3	6	0
Set Thirteen	2	4	25
Set Fourteen	1	2	0
Totals	56	112	150

CIRCUIT COURSES

Circuit training is a great way to get in shape and stay in shape. You can do this alone, but you may find it easier to get motivated if you train with a small group. At the very least, try to find one partner who shares your fitness goals.

There are several kinds of circuit courses. Fixed circuits, like the one featured in the recruit training section of this book, require equipment that can't be moved, like pull-up and dip bars. Moveable circuits utilize equipment that can be easily transported. A simplified circuit requires no equipment and can be done anywhere: on the deck of a ship, on a basketball court, in a field.

To train using a simplified circuit, after warmup, start to run in a wide circle (as wide as you can depending on your location). The designated leader (if you're by yourself, try using a stopwatch with an alarm) calls the exercises at regular intervals. For example:

Run 3 minutes, stop in place.   Then do 15 pushups.
Run 3 minutes, stop in place.   Then do 25 crunches.
Run 3 minutes, stop in place.   Then do 20 steam-engines.
Run 3 minutes, stop in place.   Then do 10 dive bomber pushups.
Run 3 minutes, stop in place.   Then do 25 crunches.

You can develop your own series of exercises from those in the Daily 16. Total duration for the circuit should be no less than 20 minutes.

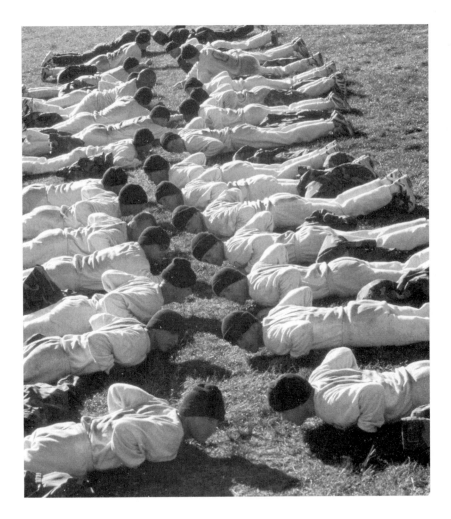

PREPARING FOR THE MARINE CORPS

The United States Marine Corps has developed guidelines for men and women to ready them for Marine Corps recruit training. These can be followed precisely or can be tailored to meet your fitness goals. Some of the exercises will be followed by numbers like 20/3. This means the exercise needs to be conducted with 20 repetitions for 3 sets (or 3 times with a short rest in between each set). If you have any questions concerning this workout check our website at www.getfitnow.com and ask your question on our bulletin board.

FOUR WEEK FITNESS PLAN

This program was orginally designed for men and women entering the Delayed Entry Program (DEP) with the anticipation of arriving at Boot Camp within 4 weeks, regardless of physical fitness. All repetitions, sets and times are minimums, but you can do more if you're capable.

WEEK # 1

MONDAY	TUESDAY	WEDNESDAY
Walk: 30 min. **Stretching:** (You can use a stretching card from the Daily 16.) **Crunches:** 30 repetitions (reps) for 2 sets **Pull-ups (men):** 1 set maximum reps **Arm Hang (women):** 15 seconds for 2 sets	**Walk:** 30 min. **Stretching** **Crunches:** 30 reps for 2 sets **Pull-ups (men):** 3 sets of 1/2 max. reps **Arm Hang (women):** 15 sec. for 2 sets	**Warmup walk:** 5 min. **Stretching** **Jog:** 1 min. Then walk 4 min. for 4 sets (20 min. total) **Cooldown walk:** 5 min. **Crunches:** 30 reps for 2 sets **Pull-ups (men):** 2 sets max reps **Arm Hang (women):** 15 sec. for 2 sets

THURSDAY	FRIDAY	SATURDAY
Warmup walk: 5 min. **Stretching** **Jog:** 1 min. Then walk 4 min. for 4 sets (20 min. total) **Cooldown walk:** 5 min. **Crunches:** 30 reps for 2 sets **Pull-ups (men):** 5 sets of 1/2 max reps **Arm Hang (women):** 15 sec. for 2 sets	**Warmup walk:** 5 min. **Stretching** **Jog:** 2 min. Then walk 3 min. for 4 sets (20 min. total) **Cooldown walk:** 5 min. **Crunches:** 30 reps for 2 sets **Pull-ups (men):** 2 sets max reps **Arm Hang (women):** 15 sec. for 2 sets	**Warmup walk:** 5 min. **Stretching** **Jog:** 2 min. Then walk 3 min. for 4 sets (20 min. total) **Cooldown walk:** 5 min. **Crunches:** 30 reps for 2 sets **Pull-ups (men):** 5 sets of 1/2 max reps **Arm Hang (women):** 15 sec. for 2 sets

WEEK # 2

MONDAY	TUESDAY	WEDNESDAY
Warmup walk: 5 min. **Stretching** **Run:** 3 min. Then walk 2 min. for 4 sets (20 min. total) **Cooldown walk:** 5 min. **Crunches:** 45 repetitions for 2 sets **Pull-ups (men):** 3 sets max reps **Arm Hang (women):** 30 seconds for 2 sets: 15 seconds for 2 sets	**Warmup walk:** 5 min. **Stretching** **Run:** 3 min. Then walk 2 min. for 4 sets (20 min. total) **Cooldown walk:** 5 min. **Crunches:** 45 reps for 3 sets **Pull-ups (men):** 6 sets of 1/2 max reps **Arm Hang (women):** 20 sec. for 6 sets	**Warmup walk:** 5 min. **Stretching** **Run:** 4 min. Then walk 1 min for 4 sets (20 min. total) **Cooldown walk:** 5 min. **Crunches:** 45 reps for 2 sets **Pull-ups (men):** 3 sets max reps **Arm Hang (women):** 30 sec. for 2 sets

THURSDAY	FRIDAY	SATURDAY
Warmup walk: 5 min. **Stretching** **Run:** 4 min. Then walk 1 min for 4 sets (20 min. total) **Cooldown walk:** 5 min. **Crunches:** 45 reps for 4 sets **Pull-ups (men):** 6 sets of 1/2 max reps **Arm Hang (women):** 20 sec. for 6 sets	**Warmup walk:** 5 min. **Stretching** **Run:** 7 min. Then walk 3 min. for 2 sets (20 min. total) **Cooldown walk:** 5 min. **Crunches:** 45 reps for 2 sets **Pull-ups (men):** 3 set max reps **Arm Hang (women):** 30 sec. for 2 sets	**Warmup walk:** 5 min. **Stretching** **Run:** 7 min. Then walk 3 min. for 2 sets (20 min. total) **Cooldown walk:** 5 min. **Crunches:** 45 reps for 3 sets **Pull-ups (men):** 6 sets of 1/2 max reps **Arm Hang (women):** 30 sec. for 3 sets

WEEK # 3

MONDAY

Warmup walk: 5 min.
Stretching
Run: 8 min. Then walk 2 min. for 2 sets (20 min. total)
Cooldown walk: 5 min.
Crunches:
60 reps for 2 sets
Pull-ups (men):
3 sets max reps
Arm Hang (women):
45 second for 2 sets

TUESDAY

Warmup walk: 5 min.
Stretching
Run: 8 min. Then walk 2 min. for 2 sets (20 min. total)
Cooldown walk: 5 min.
Crunches:
60 reps for 3 sets
Pull-ups (men):
6 sets of 1/2 max reps
Arm Hang (women):
30 sec. for 3 sets

WEDNESDAY

Warmup walk: 5 min.
Stretching
Run: 20 minutes
Cooldown walk: 5 min.
Crunches:
60 reps for 2 sets
Pull-ups (men):
3 sets max reps
Arm Hang (women):
45 sec. for 2 sets

THURSDAY

Warmup walk: 5 min.
Stretching
Run: 20 minutes
Cooldown walk:
5 min.
Crunches:
60 reps for 4 sets
Pull-ups (men):
6 sets of 1/2 max reps
Arm Hang (women):
30 sec. for 4 sets

FRIDAY

Warmup walk: 20 min.
Stretching
Crunches:
60 reps for 2 sets
Pull-ups (men):
3 sets max reps
Arm Hang (women):
45 sec. for 2 sets

SATURDAY

Warmup walk: 5 min.
Stretching
Run: 1.5 mile timed
Cooldown walk: 5 min.
Crunches:
60 reps for 3 sets
Pull-ups (men):
6 sets of 1/2 max reps
Arm Hang (women):
45 sec. for 3 sets

WEEK # 4

MONDAY	TUESDAY	WEDNESDAY
Warmup walk: 5 min. *Run:* 20 min. *Cooldown walk:* 5 min. *Crunches:* 75 reps for 2 sets *Pull-ups (men):* 3 set max reps *Arm Hang (women):* 60 sec. for 2 sets	*Warmup walk:* 30 min. *Stretching* *Crunches:* 75 reps for 3 sets *Pull-ups (men):* 6 sets of 1/2 max reps *Arm Hang (women):* 30 sec. for 4 sets	*Warmup walk:* 10 min. *Stretching* *Crunches:* 75 reps for 3 sets *Pull-ups (men):* 3 sets max reps *Arm Hang (women):* 60 sec. for 2 sets

THURSDAY	FRIDAY	SATURDAY
Warmup walk: 5 min. *Stretching* *Run:* 30 min. *Cooldown walk:* 5 min. *Crunches:* 75 reps for 2 sets *Pull-ups (men):* 6 sets of 1/2 max reps *Arm Hang (women):* 45 sec. for 2 sets	*Warmup walk:* 10 min. *Stretching* *Crunches:* 75 reps for 3 sets *Pull-ups (men):* 3 sets max reps *Arm Hang (women):* 60 sec. for 2 sets	*Warmup walk:* 30 min. *Stretching* *Crunches:* 75 reps for 3 sets *Pull-ups (men):* 6 sets of 1/2 max reps *Arm Hang (women):* 60 sec. for 3 sets

6-MONTH BEGINNER'S WORKOUT

This program was originally developed by the Marine Corps for men and women in the DEP for less than 6 months and not capable of passing crunches and pull-ups (men) or flex-arm hang (women). All repetitions, sets and times are minimums, but you can do more if you are capable.

MONTH 1

WEEKS 1 & 2

Walk 15 min.:	Mon. Wed. Fri.
Stretch:	Mon. through Sat.

WEEKS 3 & 4

Walk 20 min.:	Mon. Wed. Fri.
Stretch:	Mon. Wed. Fri. Sat.
Crunches 15/2:	Mon. Fri.

MONTH 2

WEEKS 1 & 2

Walk 30 min.:	Mon. Fri.
Stretch:	Mon. Tue. Wed. Fri. Sat.
Jog and Walk 10 min.:	Wed.
Crunches 15/2:	Mon. Wed. Fri.
Daily 16:	Mon. Fri.

WEEKS 3 & 4

Walk 30 min.:	Wed.
Stretch:	Mon. Tue. Wed. Fri. Sat.
Jog 15 min.:	Mon. Fri.
Crunches 15/3:	Mon. Wed. Fri.
Calisthenics 15/2:	Wed.
Negative pullups 5/2:	Mon. Fri.

167

MONTH 3

WEEKS 1-4

Walk 30 min.:	Wed.
Stretch:	Mon. Tue. Wed. Fri. Sat.
Jog 20 min.:	Mon. Fri.
Crunches 20/3:	Mon. Wed. Fri.
Negative pull-ups 5/2:	Mon. Fri.
Daily 16: 15/2:	Mon. Fri.
Pull-ups (men) 3/2:	Wed.
Arm Hang (women) 15+ sec./2:	Wed.

MONTH 4

WEEKS 1 & 2

Stretch:	Mon. Tue. Wed. Fri. Sat.
30 min. walk or other aerobic activity:	Wed.
Jog 25 min.:	Mon. Fri.
Crunches 25/3:	Mon. Wed. Fri.
Pull-ups (men) 3+/2:	Mon. Fri.
Arm Hang (women) 15+ sec./2:	Mon. Fri.
Negative Pull-ups 5/3:	Wed.
Daily 16: 20/2:	Mon. Fri.

WEEKS 3 & 4

30 min. walk or other aerobic activity:	Wed.
Stretch:	Mon. Tue. Wed. Fri. Sat.
Jog 25 min.:	Mon. Fri.
Crunches 20/4:	Mon. Wed. Fri.
Pull-ups (men) 3+/2:	Mon. Fri.
Arm Hang (women) 15+ sec./2:	Mon. Fri.
Negative Pull-ups 10/2:	Wed.
Daily 16: 15/3:	Wed.

6-MONTH BEGINNER'S WORKOUT, *continued*

MONTH 5

WEEKS 1 & 2

30 min. walk or other aerobic activity:	Wed.
Stretch:	Mon. Tue. Wed. Fri. Sat.
Jog 30 min.:	Mon. Fri.
Crunches 30/3:	Mon. Wed. Fri.
Pull-ups (men) 3/3:	Mon. Fri.
Arm Hang (women) 15 sec/3:	Mon. Fri.
negative pullups 10/2:	Wed.
Daily 16:	Wed.

WEEKS 3 & 4

Stretch:	Mon. Tue. Wed. Fri. Sat.
30 min. walk or other aerobic activity:	Sat.
Jog 30 min.:	Mon. Wed. Fri.
Crunches 35/2:	Mon. Wed. Fri.
Pull-ups (men) 3/3:	Mon. Wed. Fri.
Arm Hang (women) 15 sec./3:	Mon. Wed. Fri.
Daily 16: 20/3:	Wed.

6-MONTH BEGINNER'S WORKOUT, *continued*

MONTH 6

WEEKS 1 & 2

30 min.walk or other aerobic activity:	Wed.
Stretch:	Mon. Tue. Wed. Fri. Sat.
Jog 30 min.:	Mon. Fri.
Crunches 40/2:	Mon. Wed. Fri.
Pull-ups (men) 3+/ 3:	Mon. Wed. Fri.
Arm Hang (women) 15+ sec./3:	Mon. Wed. Fri.
Daily 16:	Mon. Wed. Fri.

WEEK 3

30 min.walk or other aerobic activity:	Mon.
Stretch:	Mon. Tue. Wed. Fri. Sat.
Jog 20 min.:	Wed. Fri.
Crunches 40/2:	Mon. Wed. Fri.
Pull-ups (men) 3/3:	Mon. Fri.
Arm Hang (women) 15 sec/3:	Mon. Fri.
Daily 16:	Mon. Wed. Fri.

WEEK 4

Do not do any exercises except walking and stretching during the 2 days prior to being shipped.

6-MONTH MAINTENANCE WORKOUT

This program was originally developed by the Marine Corps for men and women in the DEP for less than 6 months and capable of passing crunches and pull-ups (men) or flex-arm hang (women). As such, it is more a "maintenance" program with a "push" at the end to ready recruits for Boot Camp. All repetitions, sets and times are minimums, but you can do more if you are capable.

MONTH 1

20 min.walk or other aerobic activity:	Wed.
Stretch:	Mon. Tue. Wed. Fri. Sat.
Jog 20 min.:	Mon. Fri.
Crunches 30/3:	Mon. Wed. Fri.
Pull-ups (men) 3/2:	Mon. Wed. Fri.
Arm Hang (women) 15 sec./ 2:	Mon. Wed. Fri.

MONTH 2 to 5

30 min.walk or other aerobic activity:	Wed.
Stretch:	Mon. Tue. Wed. Fri. Sat.
Jog 30 min.:	Mon. Fri.
Crunches 40/3:	Mon. Wed. Fri.
Pull-ups (men) 3/3:	Mon. Wed. Fri.
Arm Hang (women) 15 sec./3:	Mon. Wed. Fri.
Daily 16:- 20/3:	Wed.

6-MONTH MAINTENANCE WORKOUT, *continued*

MONTH 6

WEEKS 1 & 2

30 min.walk or other aerobic activity:	Wed.
Stretch:	Mon. Tue. Wed. Fri. Sat.
Jog 30 min.:	Mon. Fri.
Crunches 40/2:	Mon. Wed. Fri.
Pull-ups (men) 3/3:	Mon. Wed. Fri.
Arm Hang (women) 15 sec./3:	Mon. Wed. Fri.
Daily 16:	Mon. Wed. Fri.

WEEK 3

30 min.walk or other aerobic activity:	Mon.
Stretch:	Mon. Tue. Wed. Fri. Sat.
Jog- 20 min.:	Wed. Fri.
Crunches 40/2:	Mon. Wed. Fri.
Pull-ups (men) 3/3:	Mon. Fri.
Arm Hang (women) 15 sec./3:	Mon. Fri.
Daily 16:	Mon. Wed. Fri.

WEEK 4

Do not do any exercises except walking and stretching during the 2 days prior to being shipped.

64-DAY BOOT CAMP WORKOUT

Want a taste of what it's really like at Boot Camp? Take a look at this authentic PT schedule from one Marine Corps Recruit Basic Training class.

KEY

TD = Training Day   SQD. ABIL. = Squad Ability Run
PT = Physical Training   SITS = Situps
FLEX = Flexibilty   PULLS = Pull-ups
TABLE = Table Exercises   O'COURSE = Obstacle Course

TD 1:   1.5 MILE FORM RUN 9 MIN. PACE/FLEX CLASS & TABLE/COMBAT HITTING SKILLS I
TD 2:   COMBAT HITTING SKILLS II
TD 3:   1.5 MILE SQD. ABIL. (MODERATE PACE) CIRCUIT COURSE/LINE I PART I (SELF-DEFENSE TRAINING)
TD 4:   COMBAT HITTING SKILLS III / INTRO TO BAYONET
TD 5:   2.0 MILE FARTLEK, MAX SET SITS/ PULLS
TD 6:   2.0 FORM. RUN 9:00 PACE/ TABLE
TD 7:   PUGIL STICKS I / LINE I PART II
TD 8:   1.5 INDIVIDUAL EFFORT RUN/ RIFLE PT/ TIMED SIT-UPS
TD 9:   NO PT
TD 10:   1.0 MILE WARMUP JOG/ O'COURSE
TD 11:   LINE I PART III
TD 12:   PUGILSTICKS II / LINE II PART I
TD 13:   2.0 MILE FORMATION RUN NFT 8:45 PACE/ CIRCUIT COURSE
TD 14:   .5 MI. WARMUP / 1.0 MI. SQD ABIL. INTER. 30/60 MAX SET SITS/ PULLS .5 MI. COOLDOWN
TD 15:   3.0 Mile March / Confidence Course
TD 16:   No PT
TD 17:   2.0 Mile Timed Run / Max Set Sits / Pulls / Line II Part II
TD 18:   2.5 Mile SQD ABIL. / TABLE / INTRO TO LOG DRILL/ PUGIL STICKS III
TD 19:   .5 MILE Warmup /1.5 MILE INTERVAL 30 / 60 / CIRCUIT COURSE
TD 20:   NO PT.
TD 21:   2.5 MILE INDIVIDUAL EFFORT/ O'COURSE/ STRETCHING
TD 22:   LINE DRILLS
TD 23:   5.0 MILE MARCH
TD 24:   COMBAT SURVIVAL SWIM I
TD 25:   2.0 MILE SQD RUN NOT FOR TIME 8:45 MIN PACE/ .5 HOUR **173**

FLEX/ COMBAT SURVIVAL SWIM II
TD 26:   COMBAT SURVIVAL SWIM III
TD 27:   3.0 MILE SQD ABILITY RUN/ CIRCUIT COURSE/ COMBAT SUR-
VIVAL SWIM IV
TD 28:   NO PT
TD 29:   2.0 MILE INTERVAL 60/ 60 ONE SET SITS AND PULLS
TD 30:   6.0 MILE NIGHT MARCH
TD 31:   NO PT
TD 32:   3.0 MI INDIVIDUAL RUN/ SITS & PULLS
TD 33:   NO PT
TD 34:   NO PT
TD 35:   CONFIDENCE COURSE
TD 36:   0.5 MILE WARMUP/ 2.5 INTERVAL / 60 60 RIFLE PT
TD 37:   NO PT
TD 38:   3.0 MILE INDIV EFFORT 75% / TIMED SITS & MAX PULLS /
STRETCHING
TD 39:   NO PT
TD 40:   PHYSICAL FITNESS TEST
TD 41:   10 MILE MARCH
TD 42:   2.0 MILE RUN INDIVIDUAL EFFORT/ RIFLE PT/ STRETCHING
TD 43:   3.0 MILE FORMATION RUN/ CIRCUIT COURSE
TD 44:   NO PT
TD 45:   NO PT
TD 46:   NO PT
TD 47:   2.0 MILE BOOTS / UTILITIES RIFLES/ O'COURSE/ FIELD   MEET
TD 48:   NO PT
TD 49:   NO PT
TD 50:   NO PT
TD 51:   3.0 MILE BOOTS & UTILITIES W/ RIFLE / O' COURSE
TD 52:   3.0 MILE SOD INDIAN RUN/ TABLE/ LOG DRILLS/ STRETCHING
TD 53:   4.0 MILE PLATOON MOTIVATION RUN/ TABLE
TD 54:   NO PT
TD 55:   NO PT
TD 56:   NO PT
TD 57:   CRUCIBLE EVENT
TD 58:   CRUCIBLE EVENT
TD 59:   9 MILE MARCH TO BATTALION AREA
TD 60:   NO PT
TD 61:   NO PT
TD 62:   NO PT
TD 63:   4.3 MILE GRAD RUN
TD 64:   NO PT

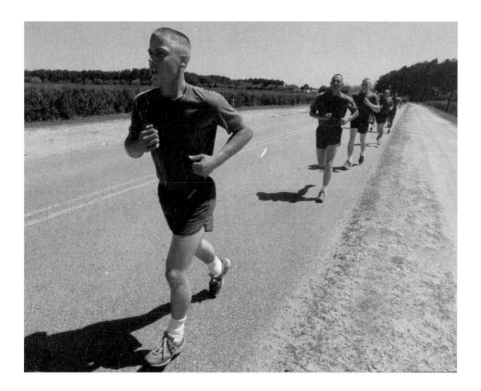

A FEW WORDS ABOUT RUNNING

Running and its milder form, jogging, are excellent ways to build your cardiovascular fitness level. Because your full body weight is supported and lifted during running and jogging, the potential for leg injuries increases. Proper running form, surface considerations, proper footwear and thorough stretching are keys to exercising comfortable and reducing injuries.

Proper Form. Proper form will help you run more efficiently. Keep your head up with a slight forward lean. Don't slouch, keep your head down, or droop your shoulders. Your head should be held upward, with your eyes focused 10 to 20 yards ahead. Use a smooth, rhythmic and relaxed arm and shoulder action. Your legs should move freely and naturally from the hips without exaggerated lifting of the knees and feet.

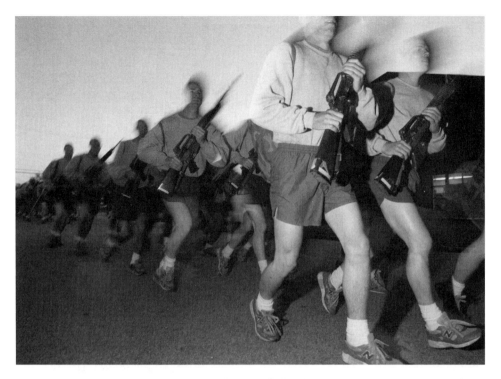

During the "recovery" phase of the leg action, as your rear foot lifts off the ground and starts forward, your foot should pass directly beneath the knee. Avoid rotating your leg outward at the hip. During the "driving" phase of the leg action, as your lead foot strikes the ground, your toes should be pointed forward.

Proper Surface. When running on roads take all safety precautions that apply to a pedestrian. Run toward traffic whenever possible. If running at night, wear reflective gear. Try to vary the surfaces you run on (asphalt, grass, dirt, etc.). Try to run on level surfaces to avoid injury, since constant exercise on hard surfaces may cause stress to the lower extremities.

Proper Clothing. Serious problems can arise if you allow your body to overheat. By perspiring, your body prevents overheating.

Evaporation of perspiration cools the skin and helps control body temperature. Covering the body retards this cooling effect. Do not wear plastic or rubber sweatsuits. They will not allow body heat to escape and the temperature of your body will continue to rise. This can be lethal! Your running clothes need to fit loosely. They should not bind or restrict your motions.

Proper Footwear. A quality shoe is the most important investment for running. The importance of selecting a good shoe for running cannot be overemphasized. Do not run in cross trainers. Keep in mind that a shoe's ability to protect you from injury decreases as its mileage increases. You should record your daily mileage and replace your running shoes every 500-700 miles, even if there is no significant visible wear.

The Marine Corps Recruit Basic Training Program issues the New Balance 497 for all incoming recruits. Obviously one shoe for 40,000 recruits may not be the best shoe for everyone. But the 497 is a high-quality, "neutral" shoe, for a neutral foot. This shoe is effective for 70 percent of the recruits. Another 25 percent of the recruits may have some type of a flat foot or lower arch. Another 5 percent may have a high arch. These recruits require special, more specific shoes.

Proper Hydration. If you interrupt your body's cooling process by covering your body and trapping perspiration, your core temperature can rise dramatically, resulting in heat exhaustion or heat stroke. Even a well-conditioned Marine can suffer heat exhaustion if unable to remove this excess heat and replace needed fluids. Drink as much as possible before, during, and after exercise. Do not take salt tablets. They only add to the problem by upsetting the body's electrolyte balance.

Failure to acclimate before a strenuous workout in the heat, especially with high humidity, invites heat injury. Adapting to a hot environment usually takes about two weeks. Individuals who are physically fit acclimate faster than those not in top physical shape.

When exercising in the sun, try to wear light (color and weight) clothing. The lighter colors will reflect the sun's rays and the lighter

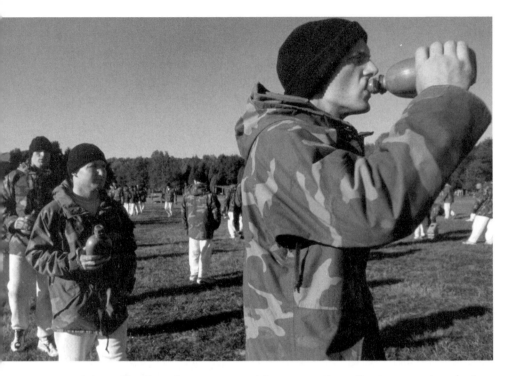

weight will allow for more rapid evaporation. Try to exercise during the coolest parts of the day (early morning or late evening). Also reduce the intensity of your exercise to decrease the heat stress on your body when it is extremely hot.

Dehydration is a constant threat when exercising in the heat. If you start to get thirsty it is too late! Drink plenty of water before, during, and after your workouts. . . before you get thirsty. Drink up to eight quarts of water a day if you are undergoing rigorous physical training.

TYPES OF HEAT INJURIES, SYMPTOMS, AND TREATMENT

Heat Cramps are the result of hard work in the heat. Heavy sweating is associated with heat cramps. Symptoms include muscular twitching or cramping and muscular spasms in the arms, legs, and abdomen.

WHAT ABOUT EXERCISING IN COLD WEATHER?

In general, cold weather conditions favor the loss of internal body heat, and as such your body will remain cool. After exercise, however, it is important to wear warmup gear. Chilling can occur rapidly as accumulated sweat clings to the body and clothing.

Here are a few simple guidelines to remember when exercising in cool and cold weather.

- Layer your clothing. Remove and replace layers as needed. Keep in mind that it's easy to get overheated, even in cold weather, so manage your layers to stay comfortable. Include a hat and gloves in your layering system.

- Ventilate your sweat. Allow sweat to evaporate from your body and clothing. If your clothes are soaking wet, chances are you'll lose body heat when you are resting. Manage those layers!

- Choose your clothing wisely. Use polypropylene (or wool) outer garments, which retain heat when wet. Avoid cotton clothing in cold weather. For an outer shell, use a garment made of material which permits sweat vapor to escape through micropores. There are many excellent synthetic materials which make for comfortable cold weather workouts.

- Drink plenty of water. Stay hydrated. It's easy to neglect this when it's cold outside, but your body needs plenty of fluids when exercising under any environmental condition.

Heat Stress may follow or occur in conjunction with heat cramps. It results from adjustments made in the circulatory system, especially the blood vessels close to the skin, to keep internal body temperature down. Symptoms include fatigue, pale skin, blurred vision, low blood pressure and dizziness. Heat stress left untreated can progress to heat exhaustion.

Heat Exhaustion occurs when heat stress is left untreated. It is caused by prolonged sweating with inadequate fluid replacement. Symptoms are excessive thirst, fatigue, lack of coordination, increased sweating, cool or wet skin and abnormally high internal body temperature.

For all of these heat injuries, the individual should be moved immediately to a cool place and given plenty of water. In the case of heat exhaustion medical attention is necessary.

Heat Stroke is a medical emergency because it is life threatening. The cause of heat stroke is a breakdown of the body's cooling mechanism. Symptoms may include little or no sweating, hot or dry skin, high internal body temperature (above 105 degrees Fahrenheit), rapid pulse, rapid breathing, coma and seizures.

Treatment of heat stroke involves cooling the body by moving the individual to a cooler location. The victim should be sponged with cool water, applying ice to the armpits, groin and back of the neck. The victim should not be immersed in cold water, because this may cause shock. Urgent medical attention is required.

HYDRATION GUIDELINES

- Begin drinking fluids before participating in any exercise activity. There is no such thing as too much water.

- Use water rather than drinks that contain sugar. Sugar interferes with the absorption process.

- Drink cool water. Studies show that cool water is absorbed from the stomach faster than water of other temperatures.

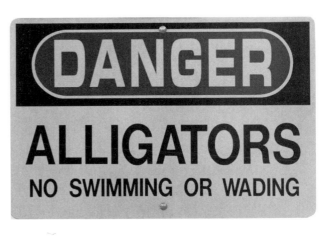

- Drink before you become thirsty. The body's thirst mechanism is about one quart behind the need.

- Do not use salt tablets. They can be very dangerous because you have no method to determine how much salt has been lost. Salt makes up a very low percent of perspiration. Too much salt can create a problem.

- Check your weight immediately following exercise. If you are working out very hard, you may lose two pounds or more. To replace this loss (which is mostly water), you should drink at least one quart of water for each two pounds of fluid lost. The replacement of lost water is very important for continued efficient exercise.

NUTRITION

Y ou can't achieve peak physical fitness without paying attention to what you eat. Strong dietary habits are critical both before entering the Marine Corps and during Marine Corps training as well. Optimum performance is achieved by proper nutrient intake and is essential to receiving maximum performance output during exercise. Nutrition also promotes vital muscle and tissue growth and repair. The ideal diet provides all the nutrients that the body needs and supplies energy for exercise.

The Navy has developed a nutrition and weight control program to enable participants to vastly improve their health and fitness. The program deals with excess body fat and highlights the foods that will be most effective in helping you achieve your personal fitness goals. Used in conjunction with this or any physical conditioning regimen, this nutrition program will help you maintain and improve your health.

The following information on nutrition is essential for adopting healthy eating and exercise habits. Although the program is designed

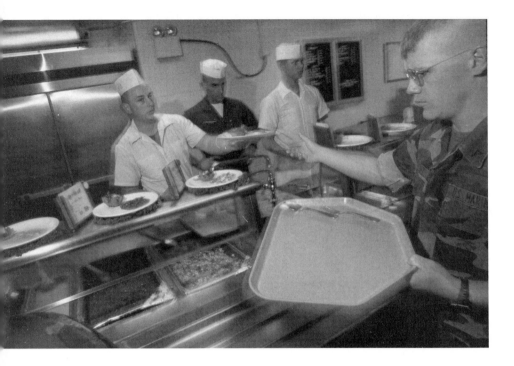

primarily as a weight management education tool, the Navy recommends it to all Marines for the maintenance of long-term optimum health. The nutrition and diet program is successful only when used in conjunction with a physical conditioning program and is not to be used as a one-time, "quick fix" diet.

For example, a weight-loss program that reduces fat and incorporates complex carbohydrates but does not include exercise will ultimately fail. Similarly, increased exercise without a carefully monitored calorie intake will bring disappointing results. You need to consume a great amount of complex carbohydrates to provide the energy you need to sustain a strenuous physical program at the Academy.

Before starting a nutrition or a weight-control program, it is essential to understand the way our bodies process the foods we eat.

WHAT IS NUTRITION?

Nutrition is the science of nourishment, the study of nutrients and the process by which organisms use them. In other words, nutrition is the way our bodies get energy from the food we eat. So the old saying,

A healthy body fat percentage for men is 14 to 16 percent; for women, 24 to 26 percent.

"You are what you eat," may not be far from the truth, considering the performance of the body is directly related to how we fuel ourselves. The study of nutrition has proven that poor nutritional habits have a profound effect on physical and mental capabilities and affect all functions of the body. Without the most fundamental of nutrients, including water, the body quickly begins to deteriorate.

Good nutrition is fundamental to every living organism on the earth in order to grow and function properly. There are six nutrients derived from food: carbohydrates, protein, and fat, which provide the body with calories; and vitamins, minerals, and water, which provide no calories. It is important to note that while carbohydrates and proteins supply the body with four calories each per gram, fat contributes nine calories per gram—more than double. Therefore, it is important to monitor fat intake when maintaining or losing weight.

After exhaustive exercise, it takes at least 20 hours to completely restore muscle energy.

Similarly, a diet and exercise program must incorporate carbohydrates that provide the body with the energy needed to sustain an exercise regimen.

Carbohydrates are sugars and starches in food and are derived from the plant kingdom. Typically, carbohydrates are called either simple or complex and provide the body with most of its fuel. Examples of complex carbohydrates include bread, rice, pasta, potatoes, cereals, and whole grains. Simple carbohydrates include fruits and vegetables. Refined simple sugars are found in candy, cakes, cookies, sodas, etc.

and provide a quick source of energy. Some carbohydrates, such as fruits and vegetables, are also rich in dietary fiber, another chief element of a healthy diet.

Dietary fiber is found only in plant food and is the "indigestible" part of the plant. So although fiber is edible, it is not digested or absorbed by humans. Similarly, fiber itself is calorie-free although typically foods rich in fiber usually contain calories. Fiber is made up of

A high carbohydrate diet is essential to maintaining energy during heavy training.

two types: soluble and insoluble. Soluble fiber lowers cholesterol levels. Its sources include fruits and vegetables, especially apples, oranges, carrots, oat bran, barley, and beans. Insoluble fiber increases the bulk of food thereby speeding the passage of food through the digestive tract. Insoluble fiber is found in fruits with edible skins, whole grains and breads, and whole grain cereals. Although 25 to 30 grams of fiber per day is recommended, statistics show that most Americans fail to consume this recommended daily allowance and take in only 10 to 15 grams per day.

Protein is essential to the human body. Protein functions to repair and build tissues, provide a structural role in all body tissues and contributes to the formation of enzymes, hormones, and antibodies. Protein consists of amino acids that are sometimes called the "building blocks" of protein. Protein in the diet is broken down into amino acids during digestion. Complete proteins are foods containing large amounts of essential amino acids. Complete proteins are found in animal proteins including beef, chicken, pork, fish, eggs, milk, and cheese. There are also incomplete proteins, which, as their name implies, are deficient in one or more of the eight essential amino acids. Incomplete proteins are derived from non-animal sources such as legumes including soybeans, peanuts, peas, beans and lentils, grains, and vegetables.

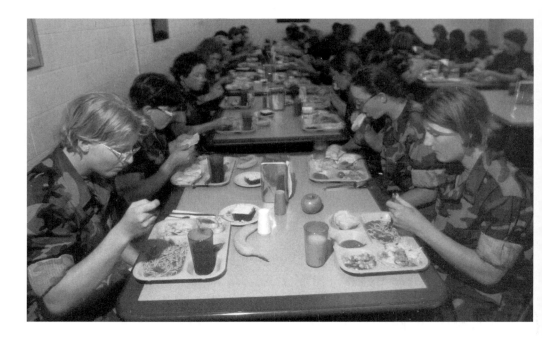

Fat. Perhaps the most talked about issue recently has been the presence of fat in our diets. Fat comes from the oils found in food and is stored in the body as triglycerides, which are more commonly known as body fat. Fat is found in vegetable oils, butter, shortening, lard, margarine, and animal foods such as beef, chicken, and diary products. The popular misconception is that all fat is bad. Adults require a minimum of 15 to 25 grams of fat daily. Fat manufactures antibodies to fight disease, serves as carriers of certain vitamins, protects vital organs, and insulates the body

The popular misconception is that all fat is bad.

against environmental temperature changes. In addition, fat lines and insulates neurons or nerves, which allow all neural information to move through the brain and the body. We would not be able to move or think without the presence of fat. There are three different kinds of fat: polyunsaturated, monosaturated, and saturated.

187

FINDING THE RIGHT BALANCE

Although conditioned to eat three meals a day, ideally we should get calories from smaller meals spread evenly throughout the day.

How does all of this translate to our personal fitness and weight loss? Remember that while carbohydrates and proteins produce only 4 calories per gram, fat provides the body with 9 calories per gram. There are 3,500 calories on one pound of fat tissue. When someone consumes 3,500 calories more than they burn, they gain one pound of fat. Similarly, when they use 3,500 calories more than they consume, they lose one pound of fat. A healthy body fat percentage for men is 14 to 16 percent; for women, 24 to 26 percent.

Although all three—carbohydrates, protein, and fat—are sources of energy nutrients, carbohydrates are the preferred source of energy for physical activity. After exhaustive exercise, it takes at least 20 hours to completely restore muscle energy, assuming that 600 grams of carbohydrates are consumed per day. A high carbohydrate diet is essential to maintaining energy during successive days of heavy training when energy stores before each training session become progressively lower.

The best sources of complex carbohydrates are bread, crackers, cereal, beans, pasta, potatoes, rice, fruits, and vegetables. *You should consume at least four servings of these food groups per day when training.*

Stay hydrated. In addition, frequent water intake is crucial. It is important to stay hydrated and consume water prior to feeling thirsty. Drink at least four quarts of water daily, staying away from alcohol, caffeine, and tobacco, which increase your body's need for water.

Good nutritional habits should not be limited to a specified training period but must become a lifetime commitment. Although we have been conditioned to think that eating three square meals per day is healthy, ideally calories should be spread evenly throughout the day with smaller meals that may occur three, four, five, or six times a day. The amount of meals and the numbers of hours in between eating should be based on each particular lifestyle.

Metabolism increases by 50 percent after eating breakfast.

Skipping meals, especially breakfast, is strongly inadvisable. According to research, approximately 90 percent of people with a weight problem skip at least one or two meals daily with breakfast being the most frequently missed. Skipping meals causes the metabolism to lower itself to conserve energy. It also promotes overeating in the evening after a meal has been skipped during the day. However, research shows that metabolism increases by 50 percent after eating breakfast.

It is strongly recommended that you keep a log of everything you have consumed, including fluids, during the day. Record each meal or snack along with the time of day. In this way, your progress will be accurately marked and serve as a vital tool in advancing your physical state of well-being.

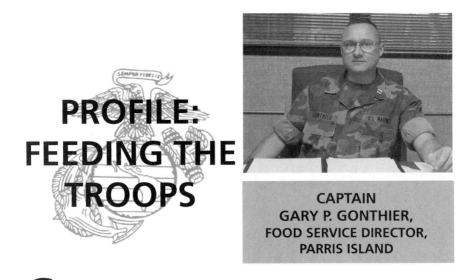

PROFILE: FEEDING THE TROOPS

**CAPTAIN
GARY P. GONTHIER,
FOOD SERVICE DIRECTOR,
PARRIS ISLAND**

Captain Gary P. Gonthier, originally from Springfield, Massachusetts, joined the Marine Corps in 1977 as an enlisted food management specialist where he was first assigned with Headquarters Battery, 3rd Marine Division in Okinawa, Japan. From there he transferred to the 8th Engineer Support Battalion in Camp Lejeune, North Carolina where he continued his work as a food service specialist. In 1979, he returned to Japan and became the Subsistence Chief in Okinawa then on to Camp Pendleton, California as the Chief Food Service Specialist.

Maintaining his position as Chief Food Service Specialist, his next several tours took him to Marine Barracks, Portsmouth Naval Shipyard in New Hampshire, then to Marine Corps Air Station Kaneohe Bay, Hawaii. In 1985, Captain Gonthier moved back to California to Camp Pendleton and then 29 Palms where he was then promoted to Food Service Operations Manager in 1989. Returning to the East Coast, Captain Gonthier worked his next tours in the Carolinas starting at Marine Corps Air Station Cherry Point in North Carolina then to Marine Corps Recruit Depot, South Carolina where he was again promoted to Food Service Director.

Currently, he is the Food Service Director at Parris Island. He holds a Bachelor of Science degree in Management from Mt. Olive, a Masters in Business from Webster University and is married with two children.

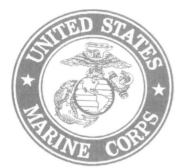

TIME PROVEN PRINCIPLES OF LEADERSHIP

Leadership principles are general rules that have guided the conduct and actions of successful leaders of the past. Although there are eleven of these principles, you will probably hear the most about the first three; be technically and tactically proficient; know yourself and seek self-improvement; and know your Marines and look out for their welfare.

Principle #1: Be technically and tactically proficient Simply stated, this principle means that you must know your job thoroughly. Try to round out your military education by going to Marine Corps schools, participating in correspondence courses through the Marine Corps Institute (MCI), and undertaking other forms of self-study. Prepare yourself for the next higher rank.

Principle #2: Know yourself and seek self-improvement. You have to know yourself in order to be a good leader, and the easiest way to do that is to sit down and honestly think about your strengths and weaknesses. Your immediate supervisor will also provide feedback on your performance. It may take many forms such as counseling, pro/con marks, and advice. Once you determine there is room for improvement, make the effort necessary to improve.

Principle #3: Know your Marines and look out for their welfare. You are probably thinking that this principle is only for those leaders senior in rank. You have to know the Marine you work with just as much as senior leaders must know their subordinates. Even as a Private or PFC in a fire team, you must know the other Marines in your team and look out for their welfare. They must do the same for you. Teamwork is the name of the game in the Corps, so make every effort to become better acquainted with your fellow Marines.

Principle #4: Keep your Marines informed. Everyone needs to know what's going on. When knowledge is shared, it encourages teamwork and enhances morale. Therefore, you should pass the word when you can.

Principle #5: Set the example Marines instinctively look to their leaders for patterns of conduct which they may either follow, emulate or use as an excuse for their own shortcomings. Others will look at the pride you show in the Corps and in being a Marine. Set the example for your fellow Marines with your personal habits. Don't use profanity just because others do. Be loyal to your seniors, peers, and subordinates. Most importantly, set the example of moral courage.

Principle #6: Ensure that the task is understood, supervised and accomplished. The leader must give clear, concise orders to avoid confusion or misunderstanding. Issuing the order is the easiest part of a leader's responsibilities. Far more important is the supervision on the leader's part to see if that order is properly executed, and the assigned task is properly performed. The leader must strike a balance between not enough supervision and too much. Too much supervision tends to destroy self-confidence, initiative and the sense of responsibility. Equally important, the subordinate is responsible to do the work without continual supervision and prompting.

Principle #7: Train your Marines as a team. You must not only know your own job but the job of the other team members as well. A unit working as a team generally gives a good account of itself. The reason is that each member is carrying his share of the load. The leader trains Marines to perform and react, to assist one another, and ensure the mission is accomplished.

Principle #8: Make sound and timely decisions. Once decisions have been made, your responsibility is to initiate action and get the job done. You should anticipate that changes may have to be made to even the best plans, so you must be prepared to adapt quickly and get on with the business at hand. You also have a responsibility to make tactful suggestions to your seniors so that they can have the best possible information upon which to base their decisions.

Principle #9: Develop a sense of responsibility in your subordinates. The lead of a unit is responsible for everything the unit does or fails to do. The leader can and should delegate authority, but can never delegate responsibility. Any effort to evade responsibility will destroy the bonds of loyalty and respect which exist between the leader and subordinates.

Principle #10: Employ your command in accordance with its capabilities. To expect a unit to do more than it is reasonably capable invites disaster. To ask it to do less is poor economics and is detrimental to accomplishing the mission. Recurrent failure may bring about a collapse of morale, esprit de corps, and efficiency. On the other hand, when the situation demands, Marines may sometimes have to be pushed far beyond their normal capabilities in order to exploit a victory or to avoid a costly defeat. Marine Corps history is abundant with examples of small units accomplishing the seemingly impossible.

Principle # 11: Take responsibility for your actions. Take initiative and look for more responsibility. Use the chain of command when you have problems or need advice. Don't get hot under the collar if someone corrects errors in your work or questions in your judgment. Accept it as valid constructive criticism and learn from it. It will help you avoid making the same mistake twice. Your leaders will be watching to see if you can handle increased responsibility, so prepare for it and be ready when they give it to you. Remember, each Marine is responsible for the effectiveness of the unit.

MARINE CORPS LEADERSHIP TRAITS

The 14 leadership traits are qualities of thought and action which, if demonstrated in daily activities, help Marines earn the respect, confidence and loyal cooperation of other Marines.

It is extremely important that you understand the meaning of each leadership trait and how to develop it, so you know what goals to set as you work to become a good leader and a good follower.

Bearing

Definition: Bearing is the way you conduct and carry yourself. Your manner should reflect alertness, competence, confidence, and control.

Suggestions for Improvement: To develop bearing, you should hold yourself to the highest standards of personal conduct. Never be content with meeting only the minimum requirements.

Courage

Definition: Courage is what allows you to remain calm while recognizing fear. Moral courage means having the inner strength to stand up for what is right and to accept blame when something is your fault. Physical courage means that you can continue to function effectively when there is physical danger present.

Suggestions for Improvement: You can begin to control fear by practicing self-discipline and calmness. If you fear doing certain things required in your daily life, force yourself to do them until you can control your reaction.

Decisiveness

Definition: Decisiveness means that you are able to make good decisions without delay. Get all the facts and weight them against each other. By acting calmly and quickly, you should arrive at a sound decision. You announce your decisions in a clear, firm, professional manner.

Suggestions for Improvement: Practice being positive in your actions instead of acting halfheartedly or changing your mind on an issue.

Dependability

Definition: Dependability means that you can be relied upon to perform your duties properly. It means that you can be trusted to complete a job. It is the willing and voluntary support of the policies and orders of the chain of command. Dependability also means consistently putting forth your best effort in an attempt to achieve the highest standards of performance.

Suggestions for Improvement: You can increase your dependability by forming the habit of being where you're supposed to be on time, by not making excuses and by carrying out every task to the best of your ability regardless of whether you like it or agree with it.

Endurance

Definition: Endurance is the mental and physical stamina that is measured by your ability to withstand pain, fatigue, stress, and hardship. For example, enduring pain during a conditioning march in order to improve stamina is crucial in the development of leadership.

Suggestions for Improvement: Develop your endurance by engaging in physical training that will strengthen your body. Finish every task to the best of your ability by forcing yourself to continue when you are physically tired and your mind is sluggish.

Enthusiasm

Definition: Enthusiasm is defined as a sincere interest and exuberance in the performance of your duties. If you are enthusiastic, you are optimistic, cheerful, and willing to accept the challenges.

Suggestions for Improvement: Understanding and belief in your mission will add to your enthusiasm for your job. Try to understand why even uninteresting jobs must be done.

Initiative

Definition: Initiative is taking action even though you haven't been given orders. It means meeting new and unexpected situations with prompt action. It includes using resourcefulness to get something done without the normal material or methods being available to you.

Suggestions for Improvement: To improve your initiative, work on staying mentally and physically alert. Be aware of things that need to be done and then do them without having to be told.

Integrity

Definition: Integrity means that you are honest and truthful in what you say and do. You put honesty, sense of duty, and sound moral principles above all else.

Suggestions for Improvement: Be absolutely honest and truthful at all times. Stand up for what you believe to be right.

Judgment

Definition: Judgment is your ability to think about things clearly, calmly, and in an orderly fashion so that that you can make good decisions.

Suggestions for Improvement: You can improve your judgment if you avoid making rash decisions. Approach problems with a common sense attitude.

Justice

Definition: Justice is defined as the practice of being fair and consistent. A just person gives consideration to each side of a situation and bases rewards or punishments on merit.

Suggestions for Improvement: Be honest with yourself about why you make a Particular decision. Avoid favoritism. Try to be fair at all times and treat all things and people in an equal manner.

Knowledge

Definition: Knowledge is the understanding of a science or art. Knowledge means that you have acquired information and that you understand people. Your knowledge should be broad, and in addition to knowing your job, you should know your unit's policies and keep up with current events.

Suggestions for Improvement: Increase your knowledge by remaining alert. Listen, observe, and find out about things you don't understand. Study field manuals and other military literature.

Loyalty

Definition: Loyalty means that you are devoted to your country, the Corps, and to your seniors, peers, and subordinates. The motto of our Corps is Semper Fidelis (Always Faithful). You owe unwavering loyalty up and down the chain of command, to seniors, subordinates, and peers.

Suggestions for Improvement: To improve your loyalty you should show your loyalty by never discussing the problems of the Marine Corps or your unit with outsiders. Never talk about seniors unfavorably in front of your subordinates. Once a decision is made and the order is given to execute it, carry out that order willingly as if it were your own.

Tact

Definition: Tact means that you can deal with people in a manner that will maintain good relations and avoid problems. It means that you are polite, calm, and firm.

Suggestions for Improvement: Begin to develop your tact by trying to be courteous and cheerful at all times. Treat others as you would like to be treated.

Unselfishness

Definition: Unselfishness means that you avoid making yourself comfortable at the expense of others. Be considerate of others. Give credit to those who deserve it.

Suggestions for Improvement. Avoid using your position or rank for personal gain, safety, or pleasure at the expense of others. Be considerate of others.

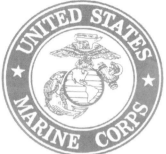

GLOSSARY OF MARINE CORPS TERMS

Aft: The rear portion of a ship

Ashore: Off station; where you go on leave or liberty

Aye Aye, Sir: Official acknowledgment of an order

Barracks: Any building where Marines live

Below: Downstairs

Bivouac: An area where you pitch tents in the field to stay overnight

Blouse: Coat

Boondocks: Woods or wilds; training area

Brightwork: Brass or shiny metal; i.e., water faucets, doorknobs, etc.

Bulkhead: Wall

Bunk or Rack: Bed

Chit: A small piece of paper; a receipt or authorization

CMC: Commandant of the Marine Corps

CO: Commander; Commanding Officer

Colors: Organizational flags; raising or lowering of the national flag

Cover: Hat

Cruise or Tour: Period of enlistment; deployment

Deck: Floor

Drill: March

Ensign: National flag

Esprit de Corps: Spirit of camaraderie

Fore: The front or forward portion of a ship

Field: Boondocks where you train
Field day: Cleaning up an area
Galley: Kitchen
Gangway: Move out of the way or make room
Gear Locker: Storage room or locker for cleaning purposes
Gung ho: Working together; in the spirit
Hatch: Door
Head: Bathroom
Ladder: Stairs
Leave: Authorized vacation
Liberty: Authorized free time, but not leave
MCRD: Marine Corps Recruit Dept; where recruits train to be Marines
MOS: Military Occupational Specialty
NCO: Noncommissioned Officer
NCOIC: Noncommissioned Officer in Charge
Overhead: Ceiling
Passageway: Corridor or hallway
Port: The left side of a ship
Porthole: Window
PFT: Physical Fitness Test
PX: Post Exchange; comparable to a civilian department store
Quarterdeck: The most revered part of a ship; where boarding and ceremonies take place
Quarters: A place to live; i.e., house, barracks, etc.
Reveille: Time to get up
Secure: Stop work, put away, close or lock
Scuttlebutt: Water fountain rumors
Snapping in: Practicing getting into firing position
Starboard: The right side of a ship
Squad bay: Large room in barracks where Marines live
Square away: Straighten up, make neat
Survey: Turn in unserviceable items
Swab: Mop
Taps: Time to sleep
Topside: Upstairs

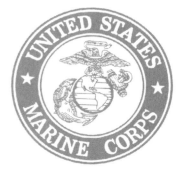

UNITED STATES MARINE CORPS RECRUITING INFORMATION

For more information about how to become a Marine, speak with your local Marine Corps Recruiter

OR CALL TOLL FREE
1- 800 - MARINES

Visit the Marine Corps Website:
www.marines.com

OR WRITE

Marine Corps Headquarters address:
United States Marine Corps Recruiting Command
2 Navy Annex
Washington, DC 20380-1775

ABOUT THE AUTHORS

ANDREW FLACH

A lifelong fitness enthusiast, Andrew was born and raised in New York City, and is a graduate of St. David's School, The Browning School, and Vassar College. When he is not running a multi-million dollar media business, his recreational pursuits include sailing, mountaineering, rock climbing, mountain biking, SCUBA diving, and flying. He still resides in New York City.

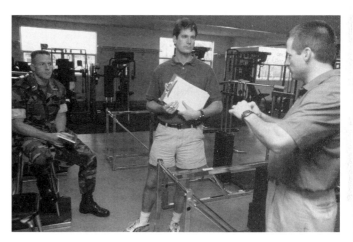

PETER FIELD PECK

Peter Field Peck is a freelance photographer. His work has appeared nationally in newspapers, magazines, and books. He currently resides in New York City.

The Complete Guide to Navy SEAL Fitness
by Stewart Smith, USN (SEAL)

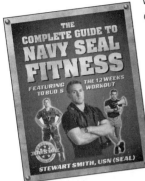

Whether you want to be a Navy SEAL or just be as fit as one...here's your chance!

Navy SEALs are ordinary people who do extraordinary jobs. It takes an optimal level of fitness to swim 6 miles, run 15 miles and perform over 150 pull-ups, 400 pushups and 400 situps in one day—but more importantly it takes motivation and determination to stick with it to the end. If you follow and finish this workout, you will find yourself in the best physical shape of your life!

Just $14.95!

plus $3.00 S/H

ISBN 1-57826-014-0

Also available on video:
The Five Star Fitness Adventure: Navy SEAL Fitness

Join Stew Smith as he shows you the proper physical fitness and conditioning techniques used by the Navy SEALs. Don't miss out on this incredible video—the swimming sequences demonstrating the combat swimmer stroke are awesome!

Featuring detailed instruction on:
- Stretching
- Running
- Upper body, lower body, and ab PT
- Pull-ups
- Swimming...and more!

Just $19.95!
plus $3.00 S/H
ISBN 1-57826-015-9

The Navy SEALs Workout Video

55 minutes of the most intense total body workout you've ever seen!

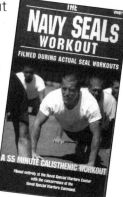

Filmed during actual SEAL workouts, this calisthenics workout is guaranteed to get you into "fighting shape" the SEAL way—by the same proven program that produces these special men trained to prevail from sea, land, or air.

The physical training is led on-camera by veteran SEAL instructors who demonstrate proper techniques and instill the special spirit and motivation to succeed for which the SEALs are renowned.

Come participate in the physical training of the most versatile, best-conditioned military unit in the world with **The Navy SEALs Workout!**

The Official United States Navy SEAL Workout

Researched by Andrew Flach
Photographed by Peter Field Peck

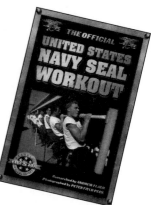

The Official United States Navy SEAL Workout presents an accurate documentation of the demanding physical training (or P.T., as it's known in military circles) that students encounter at BUD/S. The physical expectations of BUD/S graduates are awesome…but they are achievable, as this book demonstrates.

You'll learn what it's like to be a SEAL in this incredible book that brings together the fitness requirements, history, and traditions of the US Navy SEALs. Whether you're seriously into exercising or just want to start a personal fitness program, you can follow this All-American workout to strengthen and tone your entire body!

You'll find:

- Workouts you can perform at home, the gym or on the road

- Tips on stretching, lower and upper body workouts, and abdominal workouts

- Intense photos of SEALs as they prepare for missions around the world

- What it takes to become a Navy SEAL

- Full color photos of the Navy SEAL Obstacle Course…and more!

Start your workout today with the US Navy SEALs!

Just $14.95!
plus $3.00 S/H
ISBN 1-57826-007-4

To order call toll-free 1-800-906-1234